Severe Asthma

Yong Chul Lee · So Ri Kim
Seong Ho Cho

Editors

Severe Asthma

Toward Personalized Patient
Management

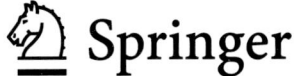 Springer

Editors
Yong Chul Lee
Department of Internal Medicine
Chonbuk National Univ. Medical School
Jeonju, Jeollabuk-do
South Korea

So Ri Kim
Department of Internal Medicine
Chonbuk National Univ. Medical School
Jeonju, Jollabuk-do
South Korea

Seong Ho Cho
Department of Internal Medicine
Morsani College of Medicine
Tampa, Florida, USA

ISBN 978-981-10-1997-5   ISBN 978-981-10-1998-2   (eBook)
https://doi.org/10.1007/978-981-10-1998-2

Library of Congress Control Number: 2017957627

Printed on acid-free paper

This Springer imprint is published by Springer Nature
The registered company is Springer Nature Singapore Pte Ltd.
The registered company address is: 152 Beach Road, #21-01/04 Gateway East, Singapore 189721, Singapore

Preface

Considerable efforts of clinicians and researchers have been concentrated to define the concept of severe asthma and to understand its pathogenesis through a multifaceted approach. Nowadays, asthma is accepted as a heterogeneous disease; is defined as a clinical syndrome of intermittent respiratory symptoms triggered by viral upper respiratory infections, environmental allergens, or other stimuli; and is characterized by nonspecific bronchial hyperresponsiveness and airway inflammation. In addition, the term "severe asthma" is based on the characteristic of resistance to the current standard treatment including inhaled steroid. Asthma heterogeneity is most easily recognized in severe asthma, where patients have diverse symptom profiles and altered responses to medications. Thus, identification of various phenotypes of severe asthma and understanding their pathogenesis are expected to provide a cornerstone to develop novel therapeutics, fulfilling the unmet needs of patients suffering from severe asthma. This book presents state-of-the-art knowledge on severe asthma, covering general information, clinical significance, pathogenesis, diagnostic modalities, and therapeutics. In particular, for readers to grasp the content easily, basic experimental data and clinical information are simultaneously provided with intuitive schematic figures. Tips on management as well as cutting-edge preclinical and clinical data of severe asthma will be very helpful for medical students, researchers, general physicians, specialists, and related paramedical staff. We hope this book can be a useful guide for your research and medical practice and understanding the changes of concept of asthma and its pathophysiology.

Jeonju, South Korea   Yong Chul Lee
Jeonju, South Korea   So Ri Kim
Tampa, FL   Seong H. Cho
May, 2017

Contents

List of Contributors

Sultan Alandijani, M.D. Division of Allergy-Immunology, Department of Internal Medicine, Morsani College of Medicine, University of South Florida, Tampa, FL, USA

Yoon-Seok Chang, M.D., Ph.D. Division of Allergy and Clinical Immunology, Department of Internal Medicine, Seoul National University Bundang Hospital, Seoul National University College of Medicine, Seongnam, South Korea

Seong H. Cho, M.D. Division of Allergy-Immunology, Department of Internal Medicine, Morsani College of Medicine, University of South Florida, Tampa, FL, USA

Mark C. Glaum, M.D., Ph.D. Division of Allergy-Immunology, Department of Internal Medicine, Morsani College of Medicine, University of South Florida, Tampa, FL, USA

Jae Seok Jeong, M.D., Ph.D. Division of Respiratory Medicine and Allergy, Department of Internal Medicine, Chonbuk National University Medical School, Jeonju, South Korea

Gong Yong Jin, M.D., Ph.D. Department of Radiology, Chonbuk National University Medical School, Jeonju, South Korea

So Ri Kim, M.D., Ph.D. Division of Respiratory Medicine and Allergy, Department of Internal Medicine, Chonbuk National University Medical School, Jeonju, South Korea

Yong Chul Lee, M.D., Ph.D. Division of Respiratory Medicine and Allergy, Department of Internal Medicine, Chonbuk National University Medical School, Jeonju, South Korea

Wenjing Li, M.D. Department of Allergy, Tongji Hospital, Wuhan, Hubei, P.R.China

Chen Hsing Lin, M.D. Division of Allergy-Immunology, Department of Internal Medicine, Morsani College of Medicine, University of South Florida, Tampa, FL, USA

Part I

Overview of Severe Asthma

Basics of Severe Asthma in Clinical Practice

1

Jae Seok Jeong and Yong Chul Lee

1.1 Definition of Severe Asthma

Bronchial asthma is now widely recognized as a heterogeneous clinical syndrome consisting of various disease phenotypes. Each asthma phenotype may have distinct observable molecular, cellular, morphological, functional, and clinical features [1, 2], all of which can be possibly integrated into specific biological mechanisms, called as endotypes [3]. Although differentiating asthma into various phenotypes/endotypes remains speculative so far, these concepts of separation may be useful in characterizing and predicting disease severity, progression, and response to general and specific therapies including biologic medications [4]. This is particularly important for severe asthma patients who are refractory to current standard therapies including inhaled and systemic corticosteroids (CS) and bronchodilators. Because these patients account for a significant proportion of health-care expenditure of asthma [5], recognizing the heterogeneous nature of asthma, especially severe asthma, may enable us to develop safe and effective phenotype-targeted biological therapies.

Importantly, appropriate clinical phenotyping of severe asthma patients, in turn, inevitably requires standardized definition of severe asthma which can be applied to a wide range of populations all over the world. There have been numerous proposed definitions for severe asthma in association with several respiratory and medical societies. It has been also referred as difficult, therapy-resistant, as well as refractory asthma. Firstly, to properly define the clinical situation of severe asthma, a prior diagnosis of asthma should be made. Then, clinical symptoms of bronchial asthma should persist despite the maximal treatment of current therapies. In general, previous studies have suggested that failure of controlling asthma symptoms despite the prescription of high-dose inhaled corticosteroids (ICS) may be a minimum requirement of definition for severe asthma, and numerous recent works have also stipulated the therapeutic level of severe asthma as those equivalent to high-dose therapies [6] (*see* Table 1.1).

The first definitions of severe asthma were proposed in 1999 and in 2000 by European Respiratory Society (ERS) [7] and American Thoracic Society (ATS) [8], respectively (*see* Table 1.1). These definitions of severe, difficult-to-treatment, or therapy-resistant asthma then were incorporated into several US and European severe asthma cohorts to further understand the pathophysiology, to improve management, and to develop novel therapy for the disease. These cohorts include Severe Asthma Research

J.S. Jeong • Y.C. Lee (✉)
Division of Respiratory Medicine and Allergy,
Department of Internal Medicine,
Chonbuk National University Medical School,
Jeonju 54907, South Korea
e-mail: leeyc@jbnu.ac.kr

Table 1.1 Definitions for severe asthma in various medical and respiratory societies

European Respiratory Society (ERS) task force in [7]	*Difficult/therapy-resistant asthma* can be defined as follows: Poorly controlled asthma with continuous requirement for short-acting β2-agonists despite delivery of a reasonable dose of inhaled corticosteroids (ICS); diagnosis on the basis of this definition can be established by means of follow-up of and care for the patient by a respiratory specialist for a period of ≥6 months

American Thoracic Society (ATS) workshop in [8]	Definition of *refractory asthma* requires one or both major criteria and two minor criteria:
	Major characteristics:
	  1. Treatment with continuous or near-continuous (≥50% of year) oral corticosteroids (CS)
	  2. Requirement for treatment with high-dose ICS
	Minor characteristics:
	  1. Requirement for daily treatment with a controller medication in addition to ICS
	  2. Asthma symptoms requiring short-acting β-agonist use on a daily or near-daily basis
	  3. Persistent airway obstruction
	  4. One or more urgent care visits for asthma per year
	  5. Three or more oral steroid "bursts" per year
	  6. Prompt deterioration with ≤25% reduction in oral or ICS dose
	  7. Near-fatal asthma event in the past

World Health Organization (WHO) in [14]	*Severe asthma* can be defined as follows:
	Uncontrolled asthma which can result in risk of frequent severe exacerbations (or death) and/or adverse reactions to medications and/or chronic morbidity (including impaired lung function or reduced lung growth in children)
	Severe asthma includes three groups, each carrying different public health messages and challenges:
	  1. Untreated severe asthma
	  2. Difficult-to-treat severe asthma
	  3. Treatment-resistant severe asthma. This group includes the following:
	• Asthma for which control is not achieved despite the highest level of recommended treatment: refractory asthma and CS-resistant asthma
	• Asthma for which control can be maintained only with the highest level of recommended treatment

ERS/ATS guidelines in [2]	Definition of *severe asthma* for patients aged ≥6 years: Asthma which requires high-dose ICS and long-acting β2-agonists [LABA] or leukotriene modifier/theophylline for the previous year or systemic CS for ≥50% of the previous year to prevent it from becoming "uncontrolled" or which remains "uncontrolled" despite this therapy Uncontrolled asthma defined as at least one of the following: • Poor symptom control: asthma control questionnaire (ACQ) consistently >1.5, asthma control test (ACT) <20 (or "not well controlled" by National Asthma Education and prevention program (NAEPP)/global initiative for asthma (GINA) guidelines) • Frequent severe exacerbations: two or more bursts of systemic CS (>3 days each) in the previous year • Serious exacerbations: at least one hospitalization, ICU stay or mechanical ventilation in the previous year • Airflow limitation: after appropriate bronchodilator withhold FEV_1 <80% predicted (in the face of reduced FEV_1/FVC defined as less than the lower limit of normal) Controlled asthma that worsens on tapering of these high doses of ICS or systemic CS (or additional biologics)
British Thoracic Society (BTS)/Scottish intercollegiate guidelines network (SIGN) guideline in [6]	*Difficult asthma* is defined as follows: Persistent symptoms and/or frequent asthma attacks despite treatment with high-dose therapies or continuous or frequent use of oral steroids High-dose therapies include (for inadequately controlled asthma on a combination of short-acting β2-agonists as required, medium-dose ICS, and an additional drug usually a LABA): • Increase the inhaled corticosteroids to high dose (adults) *or* • Add a leukotriene receptor antagonist *or* • Add a theophylline *or* • Add slow-release β2 agonist tablets, although caution needs to be used in patients already on long-acting β2 agonists *or* • Add tiotropium (adults)

Program (SARP) [9] initiated by National Heart, Lung, and Blood Institute (NHLBI) and a European Network for Understanding Mechanisms of Severe Asthma (ENFUMOSA) [10]. Although there were numerous differences regarding national health-care system, races, and socioeconomic status among each study population, clinical phenotypes of patients with severe asthma were quite similar in those studies. Subject with severe asthma were less atopic, had persistent symptoms despite high-dose controller and reliever medications, and had lower lung function with incomplete reversibility after bronchodilation [9–11]. Furthermore, diverse approaches on asthma phenotyping using more statistical methods (e.g., cluster analysis) [12] emphasized the heterogeneity of severe asthma phenotypes in these cohort populations [13].

Meanwhile, with the increasing needs of a definition of asthma severity that can be applied worldwide, the World Health Organization (WHO) published document on uniform definition of asthma severity, control, and exacerbation in 2010 [14]. In the document, it was described that components of asthma severity comprises four components: *level of control* (including current clinical control over previous 2–4 weeks and exacerbation over previous 6–12 months), *level of current treatment* (including inhalation technique and compliance), *responsiveness to treatment* (including relative insensitivity to CS and CS dependency), and *risk* (including likelihood of exacerbations, development of chronic morbidity such as progressive decline in lung function, and risk of adverse reactions from asthma medication). According to the document, severe asthma can be defined by the *level of clinical control* and *risks* as "uncontrolled asthma which can result in risk of frequent severe exacerbations (or death) and/or adverse reactions to medications and/or chronic morbidity (including impaired lung function or reduced lung growth in children)." The significance of the uniform definition of WHO is that it is applicable in all countries regardless of the availability to the current asthma medication and socioeconomic status, thereby allowing appropriate epidemiologic assessment of severe asthma worldwide (*see* Table 1.1).

The most recent definitions of severe asthma in several up-to-date guidelines resemble those of previous works in many ways (*see* Table 1.1). For instances, in the international ERS/ATS guidelines reported in 2014, severe asthma for patients aged ≥6 years is defined that asthma which requires high-dose ICS and long-acting β2-agonists [LABA] or leukotriene modifier/theophylline for the previous year or systemic CS for ≥50% of the previous year to prevent it from becoming "uncontrolled" or which remains "uncontrolled" despite this therapy [2]. In addition, British Thoracic Society (BTS)/Scottish Intercollegiate Guidelines Network (SIGN) guideline in 2016 defines difficult asthma as persistent symptoms and/or frequent asthma attacks despite treatment with high-dose therapies or continuous or frequent use of oral steroids [6]. Although there are still many different definitions for severe asthma available and difficulties in making an accurate definition for severe asthma, numerous data based on these definitions consistently demonstrate the heterogeneity of severe asthma in populations with asthma [15, 16]. Furthermore, with increasing appreciation on the heterogeneity of severe asthma, recent phenotyping of severe asthma in regard to natural history, clinical and physiological features, and underlying molecular pathobiology with predictable response to specific therapy have made the precision medicine possible. For example, newer guidelines recommend anti-interleukin (IL)-5 monoclonal antibody particularly in adults and adolescents (≥12 years) with severe eosinophilic asthma [2, 17]. Indeed, these conceptual advancements reflect the beginning of the new era in severe asthma management according to phenotype/endotype-driven approaches.

1.2 Epidemiology and Clinical Significance of Severe Asthma

Bronchial asthma is a major health problem all over the world, affecting 1–18% of the population in different countries [17]. It is estimated that approximately 300 million people have asthma globally including nearly 26 million asthmatic patients in the USA [18]. In real life, bronchial asthma may be associated millions of lost school and work days, long-term controller medication, regular and urgent health-care utilization, and significant comorbidities. Accordingly, annual economic burden of the bronchial asthma is reported to be about 56 billion dollars in the USA [19]. In this regard, severe asthma has growingly become major concern as it accounts for a disproportionately large proportion of asthma-associated health-care expenditures, while representing only a minority of total patients with asthma.

The exact prevalence of severe asthma is still unclear partly owing to the inhomogeneity in the definition and patient characteristics with different age, sex, race, and regional profiles across many population studies. For example, whereas the prevalence of severe asthma, defined strictly as the disease remains uncontrolled despite addressing and removing all possible factors that might aggravate the underlying disease, was shown to be only 3.6% among total asthmatics in the population study from the Netherlands [20], the prevalence of severe asthma according to the definition from the Global Initiative for Asthma (GINA) guidelines in Sweden was reported to be as high as 17.8% of adult asthmatics [21]. Despite these inconclusive results from numerous population studies, experts generally regard that severe asthma is a rare disease entity and estimated prevalence of severe asthma might be up to 5–10% of adult patients with asthma.

Furthermore, there is limited information regarding the exact disease burden and health outcomes of severe asthma to date. The Epidemiology and Natural History of Asthma: Outcomes and Treatment Regimens (TENOR) study, initiated in 2001, was a multicenter observational cohort study which primarily aimed to collect data to evaluate the natural history of severe or difficult-to-treat asthma. In this study, inclusion of severe or difficult-to-treat asthma patients was based on the physician's assessment of asthma severity and additional criteria determined by the frequency of urgent care visits and/or the use of multiple controller medica-

tions [22]. Results of the TENOR study showed that severe or difficult-to-treat asthma, regardless of age, was associated with evidently high rates of health-care use despite the use of multiple long-term controller medications. For instance, at the time of enrollment, more than 50% of patients were on three or more long-term controller medications [23]. However, 52.8% of adults (≥18 years of age), 43.6% adolescents (13–17 years of age), and 53.4% of children (6–12 years of age) reported a corticosteroid burst (short courses of corticosteroid therapy) in the 3 months before the enrollment. In addition, 15.2% of adults, 19.1% of adolescent, and 25.5% of children reported an emergency department visit in the 3 months before the baseline [22]. Similarly, in the SARP, another large cohort of severe asthma in which primary goal was to characterize subject with severe asthma to understand pathophysiologic mechanisms of the disease, severe asthma patients were older with longer disease duration, more daily symptoms, urgent health-care utilization especially intensive care, and comorbidities such as sinopulmonary infections compared to non-severe asthma [9]. In fact, substantial differences exist between two studies. Firstly, the definition of severe or difficult-to-treat asthma differs from each other. While SARP adopted the definition of severe asthma from ATS Workshop in 2000 [8], physicians were not instructed to use specific guidelines and independently assessed severity of asthma in TENOR study. Secondly, SARP included all asthma severities, whereas approximately 96% of the cohort in TENOR study was considered to have difficult-to-treat asthma based on the need for multiple drugs, occurrence of frequent and severe exacerbations, inability to avoid triggers, and complex treatment regimens [24]. Nevertheless, the similar results from these two large cohorts emphasize the medical burden of severe asthma and thus the urgent need of novel therapeutic approaches.

Another significance of TENOR is that it involves quite a large number of populations over 4000 patients, and thus numerous subgroups having different clinical phenotypes can be identified. For example, patients with aspirin sensitivity are associated with increased disease severity and, possibly, remodeling of the lower airways [25]. Moreover, one of TENOR analyses found that persistent airflow limitation (defined as post-bronchodilator FEV_1/FVC ratio of $\leq 70\%$ at two annual consecutive visits) in patients with severe or difficult-to-treat asthma is highly prevalent up to 60% and is related to several clinical and demographic factors, including older age, male, black ethnicity, current or past smoking, aspirin sensitivity, and longer duration of asthma [26]. In another analysis, increased weight is associated with worse asthma-related outcomes (e.g., poorer disease control, worse quality of life, and greater need for oral corticosteroids bursts) [27], and female patients with IgE-mediated allergic asthma are worse than the disease of male in terms of disease severity, quality of life, health-care use, disease control, and allergic comorbidities [28]. Taken together, heterogeneous nature of severe or difficult-to-treat asthma demonstrated in TENOR study, along with the similar findings in SARP [16], highlight that identification of important severe asthma phenotypes may reduce the burden of the disease and improve severe asthma-related health outcomes through phenotype-targeted therapeutic approaches.

However, physicians should be aware of numerous comorbidities and confounders that can change asthma phenotypes before commencing phenotype-based approaches in severe asthma, although there has been substantial advancement in identifying phenotypes through less biased and more statistically based methodology [1] (*see* Table 1.2).

Current smoking or exposure to second-hand smoke may be associated with the corticosteroid-resistant inflammatory process in the lung, thereby making asthma more difficult-to-treatment [29]. Moreover, environmental tobacco smoke exposure on asthmatic individuals has been reported to be associated with lower lung function and quality of life and greater risk for exacerbation, health-care use, and airway hyperresponsiveness, thereby leading to adverse asthma-related outcomes [30].

Table 1.2 Comorbidities and confounders that may impact on phenotypes of severe asthma

History of smoking or second-hand smoke

Environmental exposures: molds, viruses, bacteria, and ozone

Occupational exposures

Hormonal influences: premenstrual, menarche, menopause, pregnancy, and thyroid disorders

Obesity

Obstructive sleep apnea

Rhinosinusitis/nasal polyps

Vocal cord dysfunction

Gastroesophageal reflux disease

Psychological factors: personality trait, symptom perception, anxiety, and depression

Drugs: nonsteroidal anti-inflammatory drugs, β-adrenergic blockers, and angiotensin-converting enzyme inhibitors

Nonadherence to treatment and poor inhaler technique

Early-life exposures to diverse pathogenic microbes including molds, viruses, and bacteria may also relate to severe asthma. Particularly, fungal exposure has been reported to be associated with the development [31] and exacerbation of bronchial asthma [32–35]. Furthermore, epidemiologic studies have shown that fungal sensitization is found more often in asthmatic patients with increasing severity, and fungal sensitivity is a possible precipitating factor for life-threatening asthma [36–38]. Based on these knowledges, severe asthma with fungal sensitization (SAFS) has been proposed to investigate a particular phenotype of severe asthma with therapeutic implications in clinical trials [39]. Notably, several recent guidelines of severe asthma recommend allergen testing to molds in patients with difficult asthma and recurrent hospital admission [6]. In addition, viral and bacterial exposure may predispose susceptible individuals to initiate and exacerbate allergic inflammation in the lung [40].

Occupational exposure to various chemicals and compounds is also known to initiate and worsen asthma in susceptible patients [41], and changes in the level of female sex hormones and thyroid hormones may impact on clinical course of bronchial asthma [42]. Other common comorbidities of severe asthma include obesity, obstructive sleep apnea, rhinosinusitis/nasal polyps, vocal cord dysfunction, gastroesophageal reflux disease, and psychologic problems such as anxiety and depression, all of which can change clinical manifestation of severe asthma. Lastly, patient's adherence to the treatment and concurrent use of other medications targeting coexisting disorders such as nonsteroidal anti-inflammatory drugs, β-adrenergic blockers, and angiotensin-converting enzyme inhibitors may modify the observable characteristics of severe asthma.

1.3 Specific Considerations in Severe Asthma

1.3.1 Fungal Sensitization/Allergy-Associated Clinical Conditions

Respiratory fungal exposure is constant in humans, and fungal spores constitute the largest proportion of aerobiological particles in usual air environment [43]. Similarly, impact of respiratory fungal exposure on the clinical courses of bronchial asthma has been widely reported in the literatures for a long time [39], and fungal exposure has long been regarded as a precipitating factor for severe asthma phenotype. For example, inhalation of environmental fungal spores also led to the exacerbation of bronchial asthma control illustrated by daily variation in the patient symptoms, aggravation of the underlying pulmonary function (e.g., variations in peak expiratory flow), and increased incidence for critical events such as hospital admission and asthma-related deaths [32–35].

Furthermore, fungi can colonize, actively germinate, and infect the human respiratory tract. Moreover, they can produce a wide array of enzymes and toxins closely implicated in pathologic process such as allergic inflammation [44]. Therefore, fungi can potently sensitize and induce host immune response, in contrast to other inhalable aeroallergens such as house dust mites (HDMs), animal dander, and grass pollen [39, 45]. Consistent with this knowledge, over 50% of patients with severe asthma may be sensitized to one or more fungi [46], and, particularly, *Aspergillus fumigatus* and *Alternaria alternata*

are common airborne fungi implicated in severe asthma [39, 47]. Numerous epidemiologic studies have also demonstrated that fungal sensitization is found more often in asthmatic patients with increasing severity, and fungal sensitivity is a possible precipitating factor for life-threatening asthma [36–38].

In general, fungal sensitization/allergy-associated conditions refer to exaggerated immune responses against non-pathogenic fungi, which are mainly orchestrated by IgE and type 2 helper T (T_H2) cells. In contrast, the term of fungal infection can be applied when there is evidence of tissue dysfunction directly associated with the growth and invasion of pathogenic fungi in the host. There are several important disease entities that represent severe end of the fungal sensitization/allergy-associated conditions, including allergic bronchopulmonary aspergillosis (ABPA)/allergic bronchopulmonary mycosis (ABPM) and SAFS (*see* Table 1.3) [48]. Whereas ABPA was firstly reported in 1952, the definition of SAFS was introduced in 2006 [39] and has been used in clinical trial settings to demonstrate the possible role of antifungal therapy for treating a particular phenotype of severe asthma associated with fungi [49]. Historically, early data on fungal allergy were mainly derived from researches of ABPA/ABPM. However, ABPA/ABPM may be a severe end of the spectrum of allergic inflammation against fungi that are often associated with

Table 1.3 Definitions of ABPA/ABPM and SAFS

Disease entity	Definition
ABPA/ABPM	Asthma or cystic fibrosis (often that are not well controlled) Elevated total serum IgE (> 1000 IU/ml) Elevated IgE and/or IgG antibodies Immediate skin test positive Serum eosinophilia (> 1000 cells/μl) Presence of central (or proximal) bronchiectasis Radiographic pulmonary infiltrates
SAFS	Severe asthma Elevated total serum IgE (< 1000 IU/ml) Sensitization to any fungus by skin prick test or specific IgE

airway destruction in the later course of the disease. Thus, most patients sensitized to fungi without convincing evidence of lung damage could not have been properly incorporated into specific disease entity [48]. Thereafter, researchers have proposed SAFS that can be defined as patients having both severe asthma and evidence for fungal sensitization (i.e., positive skin prick test, positive fungal-specific IgE in blood) without satisfying the criteria of ABPA [39]. Notably, several subsequent clinical studies demonstrated the role of antifungal agents in the treatment of SAFS patient group [49, 50]. However, whereas the definition of SAFS is convenient for the patient inclusion in clinical trial settings, there are still several problems. For instance, there are conflicting results regarding the effectiveness of antifungal agents in the treatment of SAFS [51]. These results may be in part owing to the limitation in SAFS definition itself, which doesn't represent direct causality of fungal sensitization in inducing severe asthma, and the absence of standardized testing tools for fungal allergy. Further in-depth future researches on the role and involved mechanism of fungi in the pathogenesis of severe allergic lung inflammation should be warranted to develop more precise nomenclature system in fungal sensitization/allergy-associated conditions.

1.4 Conditions Mimicking Severe Asthma

Because clinical diagnosis of bronchial asthma is largely based on several parameters related to patient's respiratory symptoms and physiologic abnormalities, which are relatively nonspecific with lack of reproducibility, bronchial asthma may be mistaken for many clinical conditions inducing symptoms associated with airways obstruction (*see* Table 1.4). In particular, several disorders including vocal cord dysfunction (VCD) and ABPA may mimic or coexist with severe asthma. Thus, clinicians should consider these diseases or other possible diagnoses when a patient with a presumed diagnosis of bronchial asthma inadequately responds to asthma medication.

Table 1.4 Conditions mimicking severe asthma

Diagnoses that may masquerade as severe asthma in adults
Vocal cord dysfunction
Tracheobronchomalacia
Tumors in central airways
Relapsing polychondritis involving tracheal cartilage
Obstructive sleep apnea
Bronchiectasis
Allergic bronchopulmonary aspergillosis
Tuberculosis
Chronic obstructive pulmonary disease (COPD)
Cystic fibrosis
Tuberculosis
Obliterative bronchiolitis
Eosinophilic lung diseases
Hypersensitivity pneumonitis
Exercise-induced bronchoconstriction
Congestive heart failure

VCD, also referred as paroxysmal vocal fold motion, is one of the important mimics of severe asthma. Characteristic intermittent abnormal adduction of the vocal cord during respiration can establish the diagnosis of VCD. Patients with VCD often manifest stridor, wheezing, hoarseness, frequent cough, and shortness of breath; however, the diagnosis of VCD is quite challenging because these symptoms are frequently intermittent. Furthermore, previous reports have demonstrated that more than 70% of asthmatics have VCD simultaneously [52]. Numerous causes of VCD have been suggested including psychiatric disorders (e.g., depression and anxiety disorders), exercise, and irritants. Currently, there is no specific therapeutic agent for VCD, and patients are often referred to exercise therapies for long-term management.

ABPA is a complex hypersensitivity reaction that often occurs in patients with asthma (2–32% of asthmatics) or cystic fibrosis when bronchi become colonized by *Aspergillus* species (mostly *Aspergillus fumigatus*) [53, 54]. ABPA patients often manifest poorly controlled underlying asthma and recurrent pulmonary infiltrates. Generally, the diagnosis of ABPA is a composite of clinical, radiological, and immunologic features. In the later courses of ABPA, repeated episodes of bronchial obstruction, inflammation, and mucoid impaction can lead to irreversible structural and functional changes. Many patients with ABPA respond well to treatment with systemic corticosteroids, whereas some patients are poorly controlled by conventional management and may be complicated by progression to bronchiectasis and pulmonary fibrosis [55]. Antifungal agents such as itraconazole or voriconazole are reserved for ABPA patients with corticosteroid resistance.

References

1. Wenzel SE. Asthma phenotypes: the evolution from clinical to molecular approaches. Nat Med. 2012;18(5):716–25.
2. Chung KF, Wenzel SE, Brozek JL, Bush A, Castro M, Sterk PJ, et al. International ERS/ATS guidelines on definition, evaluation and treatment of severe asthma. Eur Respir J. 2014;43(2):343–73.
3. Lötvall J, Akdis CA, Bacharier LB, Bjermer L, Casale TB, Custovic A, et al. Asthma endotypes: a new approach to classification of disease entities within the asthma syndrome. J Allergy Clin Immunol. 2011;127(2):355–60.
4. Fajt ML, Wenzel SE. Asthma phenotypes and the use of biologic medications in asthma and allergic disease: the next steps toward personalized care. J Allergy Clin Immunol. 2015;135(2):299–310.
5. Barnes PJ. Severe asthma: advances in current management and future therapy. J Allergy Clin Immunol. 2012;129(1):48–59.
6. The 2016 BTS/SIGN British guideline on the management of asthma. https://www.brit-thoracic.org.uk
7. Chung KF, Godard P, Adelroth E, Ayres J, Barnes N, Barnes P, et al. Difficult/therapy-resistant asthma: the need for an integrated approach to define clinical phenotypes, evaluate risk factors, understand pathophysiology and find novel therapies. ERS task force on difficult/therapy-resistant asthma. European Respiratory Society. Eur Respir J. 1999;13(5):1198–208.
8. Proceedings of the ATS workshop on refractory asthma: current understanding, recommendations, and unanswered questions. American Thoracic Society. Am J Respir Crit Care Med 2000;162(6):2341–2351.
9. Moore WC, Bleecker ER, Curran-Everett D, Erzurum SC, Ameredes BT, Bacharier L, et al. Characterization of the severe asthma phenotype by the National Heart, Lung, and Blood Institute's severe asthma research program. J Allergy Clin Immunol. 2007;119(2):405–13.
10. The ENFUMOSA cross-sectional European multicentre study of the clinical phenotype of chronic severe asthma. European Network for Understanding Mechanisms of Severe Asthma. Eur Respir J 2003;22(3):470–477.
11. Kupczyk M, Wenzel S. U.S. and European severe asthma cohorts: what can they teach us about severe asthma? J Intern Med. 2012;272(2):121–32.
12. Haldar P, Pavord ID, Shaw DE, Berry MA, Thomas M, Brightling CE, et al. Cluster analysis and clinical asthma phenotypes. Am J Respir Crit Care Med. 2008;178(3):218–24.
13. Jarjour NN, Erzurum SC, Bleecker ER, Calhoun WJ, Castro M, Comhair SA, et al. Severe asthma: lessons learned from the National Heart, Lung, and Blood Institute severe asthma research program. Am J Respir Crit Care Med. 2012;185(4):356–62.
14. Bousquet J, Mantzouranis E, Cruz AA, Aït-Khaled N, Baena-Cagnani CE, Bleecker ER, et al. Uniform definition of asthma severity, control, and exacerbations: document presented for the World Health Organization consultation on severe asthma. J Allergy Clin Immunol. 2010;126(5):926–38.
15. Wu W, Bleecker E, Moore W, Busse WW, Castro M, Chung KF, et al. Unsupervised phenotyping of severe asthma research program participants using expanded lung data. J Allergy Clin Immunol. 2014;133(5):1280–8.
16. Moore WC, Meyers DA, Wenzel SE, Teague WG, Li H, Li X, et al. Identification of asthma phenotypes using cluster analysis in the severe asthma research program. Am J Respir Crit Care Med. 2010;181(4):315–23.
17. Global Strategy for Asthma Management and Prevention (2016 update). www.ginasthma.org
18. American Lung Association, http://www.lung.org/lung-health-and-diseases/lung-disease-lookup/asthma/learn-about-asthma/impact-of-asthma.html accessed April 5, 2017.
19. Lang DM. Severe asthma: epidemiology, burden of illness, and heterogeneity. Allergy Asthma Proc. 2015;36(6):418–24.
20. Hekking PP, Wener RR, Amelink M, Zwinderman AH, Bouvy ML, Bel EH. The prevalence of severe refractory asthma. J Allergy Clin Immunol. 2015;135(4):896–902.
21. Mincheva R, Ekerljung L, Bjerg A, Axelsson M, Popov TA, Lundbäck B, et al. Frequent cough in unsatisfactory controlled asthma--results from the population-based West Sweden asthma study. Respir Res. 2014;15:79.
22. Chipps BE, Zeiger RS, Borish L, Wenzel SE, Yegin A, Hayden ML, et al. Key findings and clinical implications from the epidemiology and natural history of asthma: outcomes and treatment regimens (TENOR) study. J Allergy Clin Immunol. 2012;130(2):332–42.
23. Dolan CM, Fraher KE, Bleecker ER, Borish L, Chipps B, Hayden ML, et al. Design and baseline characteristics of the epidemiology and natural history of asthma: outcomes and treatment regimens (TENOR) study: a large cohort of patients with severe

or difficult-to-treat asthma. Ann Allergy Asthma Immunol. 2004;92(1):32–9.

24. Miller MK, Johnson C, Miller DP, Deniz Y, Bleecker ER, Wenzel SE, TENOR Study Group. Severity assessment in asthma: an evolving concept. J Allergy Clin Immunol. 2005;116(5):990–5.

25. Mascia K, Haselkorn T, Deniz YM, Miller DP, Bleecker ER, Borish L, TENOR Study Group. Aspirin sensitivity and severity of asthma: evidence for irreversible airway obstruction in patients with severe or difficult-to-treat asthma. J Allergy Clin Immunol. 2005;116(5):970–5.

26. Lee JH, Haselkorn T, Borish L, Rasouliyan L, Chipps BE, Wenzel SE. Risk factors associated with persistent airflow limitation in severe or difficult-to-treat asthma: insights from the TENOR study. Chest. 2007;132(6):1882–9.

27. Haselkorn T, Fish JE, Chipps BE, Miller DP, Chen H, Weiss ST. Effect of weight change on asthma-related health outcomes in patients with severe or difficult-to-treat asthma. Respir Med. 2009;103(2):274–83.

28. Lee JH, Haselkorn T, Chipps BE, Miller DP, Wenzel SE, Tenor Study Group. Gender differences in IgE-mediated allergic asthma in the epidemiology and natural history of asthma: outcomes and treatment regimens (TENOR) study. J Asthma. 2006;43(3):179–84.

29. Marwick JA, Caramori G, Stevenson CS, Casolari P, Jazrawi E, Barnes PJ, et al. Inhibition of PI3Kdelta restores glucocorticoid function in smoking-induced airway inflammation in mice. Am J Respir Crit Care Med. 2009;179(7):542–8.

30. Comhair SA, Gaston BM, Ricci KS, Hammel J, Dweik RA, Teague WG, et al. Detrimental effects of environmental tobacco smoke in relation to asthma severity. PLoS One. 2011;6(5):e18574.

31. Harley KG, Macher JM, Lipsett M, Duramad P, Holland NT, Prager SS, et al. Fungi and pollen exposure in the first months of life and risk of early childhood wheezing. Thorax. 2009;64(4):353–8.

32. Salvaggio J, Seabury J, Schoenhardt FA. New Orleans asthma. V. Relationship between Charity Hospital asthma admission rates, semiquantitative pollen and fungal spore counts, and total particulate aerometric sampling data. J Allergy Clin Immunol. 1971;48(2):96–114.

33. Neas LM, Dockery DW, Burge H, Koutrakis P, Speizer FE. Fungus spores, air pollutants, and other determinants of peak expiratory flow rate in children. Am J Epidemiol. 1996;143(8):797–807.

34. Delfino RJ, Zeiger RS, Seltzer JM, Street DH, Matteucci RM, Anderson PR, et al. The effect of outdoor fungal spore concentrations on daily asthma severity. Environ Health Perspect. 1997;105(6):622–35.

35. Targonski PV, Persky VW, Ramekrishnan V. Effect of environmental molds on risk of death from asthma during the pollen season. J Allergy Clin Immunol. 1995;95(5 Pt 1):955–61.

36. Zureik M, Neukirch C, Leynaert B, Liard R, Bousquet J. Neukirch F; European Community respiratory health survey. Sensitisation to airborne moulds and severity of asthma: cross sectional study from European Community respiratory health survey. BMJ. 2002;325(7361):411–4.

37. O'Driscoll BR, Hopkinson LC, Denning DW. Mold sensitization is common amongst patients with severe asthma requiring multiple hospital admissions. BMC Pulm Med. 2005;5:4.

38. Black PN, Udy AA, Brodie SM. Sensitivity to fungal allergens is a risk factor for life-threatening asthma. Allergy. 2000;55(5):501–4.

39. Denning DW, O'Driscoll BR, Hogaboam CM, Bowyer P, Niven RM. The link between fungi and severe asthma: a summary of the evidence. Eur Respir J. 2006;27(3):615–26.

40. Gern JE. The ABCs of rhinoviruses, wheezing, and asthma. J Virol. 2010;84(15):7418–26.

41. Maestrelli P, Boschetto P, Fabbri LM, Mapp CE. Mechanisms of occupational asthma. J Allergy Clin Immunol. 2009;123(3):531–42.

42. van den Berge M, Heijink HI, van Oosterhout AJ, Postma DS. The role of female sex hormones in the development and severity of allergic and non-allergic asthma. Clin Exp Allergy. 2009;39(10):1477–81.

43. Twaroch TE, Curin M, Valenta R, Swoboda I. Mold allergens in respiratory allergy: from structure to therapy. Allergy Asthma Immunol Res. 2015;7(3):205–20.

44. Millien VO, Lu W, Shaw J, Yuan X, Mak G, Roberts L, et al. Cleavage of fibrinogen by proteinases elicits allergic responses through toll-like receptor 4. Science. 2013;341(6147):792–6.

45. Agarwal R. Severe asthma with fungal sensitization. Curr Allergy Asthma Rep. 2011;11(5):403–13.

46. O'Driscoll BR, Powell G, Chew F, Niven RM, Miles JF, Vyas A, et al. Comparison of skin prick tests with specific serum immunoglobulin E in the diagnosis of fungal sensitization in patients with severe asthma. Clin Exp Allergy. 2009;39(11):1677–83.

47. Knutsen AP, Bush RK, Demain JG, Denning DW, Dixit A, Fairs A, et al. Fungi and allergic lower respiratory tract diseases. J Allergy Clin Immunol. 2012;129(2):280–91.

48. Denning DW, Pashley C, Hartl D, Wardlaw A, Godet C, Del Giacco S, et al. Fungal allergy in asthma-state of the art and research needs. Clin Transl Allergy. 2014;4:14.

49. Denning DW, O'Driscoll BR, Powell G, Chew F, Atherton GT, Vyas A, et al. Randomized controlled trial of oral antifungal treatment for severe asthma with fungal sensitization: the fungal asthma sensitization trial (FAST) study. Am J Respir Crit Care Med. 2009;179(1):11–8.

50. Chishimba L, Niven RM, Cooley J, Denning DW. Voriconazole and posaconazole improve asthma severity in allergic bronchopulmonary aspergillosis and severe asthma with fungal sensitization. J Asthma. 2012;49(4):423–33.

51. Agbetile J, Bourne M, Fairs A, Hargadon B, Desai D, Broad C, et al. Effectiveness of voriconazole in the treatment of Aspergillus fumigatus-associated asthma (EVITA3 study). J Allergy Clin Immunol. 2014;134(1):33–9.

52. Parsons JP, Benninger C, Hawley MP, Philips G, Forrest LA, Mastronarde JG. Vocal cord dysfunction: beyond severe asthma. Respir Med. 2010;104(4):504–9.

53. Agarwal R, Aggarwal AN, Gupta D, Jindal SK. Aspergillus hypersensitivity and allergic bronchopulmonary aspergillosis in patients with bronchial asthma: systematic review and meta-analysis. Int J Tuberc Lung Dis. 2009;13(8):936–44.

54. Agarwal R. Allergic bronchopulmonary aspergillosis. Chest. 2009;135(3):805–26.

55. Vlahakis NE, Aksamit TR. Diagnosis and treatment of allergic bronchopulmonary aspergillosis. Mayo Clin Proc. 2001;76(9):930–8.

Chen Hsing Lin, Sultan Alandijani,
and Seong H. Cho

2.1 Asthma-COPD Overlap Syndrome and Smoking Asthmatics in Severe Asthma

Asthma, a heterogeneous disease, can occur in both pediatric and adult population. Compared to pediatric asthma in which infectious and allergic components play a major role in pathogenesis, adult asthma has more indistinct and complicated disease pathophysiology and, thus, shows a more refractory disease course and less responsiveness to treatments. Cigarette smoking, one of the other common disease modifying factors in adult asthma, can result in the development of another obstructive airway disease known as chronic obstructive pulmonary disease (COPD). After the age of 40, the diagnosis of COPD becomes prevalent, and the border between asthma and COPD starts to fade away [1, 2]. It is not uncommon to have patients who have diagnoses and/or features of both asthma and COPD, and they experience more frequent exacerbations, rapid decline in pulmonary function, poor quality of life, and high mortality than isolated asthma or COPD patients [3, 4]. Therefore, understanding "asthma-COPD overlap syndrome" (ACOS) will help to deliver precision medicine to this subpopulation of severe asthmatics.

To comprehend ACOS, it would be best to start familiarizing with these two different diseases, asthma and COPD.

2.1.1 Definition

The definition of ACOS has been very difficult to develop. The current clinical description of ACOS from a document by Global Initiative for Asthma and Global Initiative for Chronic Obstructive Lung Disease in 2015 states that "ACOS is characterized by persistent airflow limitation with several features usually associated with asthma and several features usually associated with COPD. ACOS is therefore identified in clinical practice by the features that it shares with both asthma and COPD" [5]. It also indicates that "A specific definition for ACOS cannot be developed until more evidence is available about its clinical phenotypes and underlying mechanisms" [5].

One of the major obstacles to define ACOS is not about ACOS itself but to accurately define asthma and COPD. Same with ACOS, both asthma and COPD are heterogeneous diseases. In order to cover their different phenotypes/endotypes, the current definition of both asthma and COPD has been far away from its ideal or "pure" scenarios and leaned toward to real patients [6, 7]. In addition, characteristics once thought to be specific to asthma or COPD are proven to be untrue. For

C.H. Lin • S. Alandijani • S.H. Cho (✉)
Division of Allergy-Immunology, Department of
Internal Medicine, Morsani College of Medicine,
University of South Florida, Tampa, FL 33612, USA
e-mail: scho2@health.usf.edu

© Springer Nature Singapore Pte Ltd. 2018
Y.C. Lee et al. (eds.), *Severe Asthma*, https://doi.org/10.1007/978-981-10-1998-2_2

instance, fixed airway obstruction, bronchial hyper responsiveness, airway reversibility, and chronic inflammation pattern, all the above elements cannot be used to distinguish between asthma and COPD [8]. Even bronchoscopic lung tissue biopsies obtained from both clinically typical asthma and COPD patients, reviewing pathologists have often failed to differentiate between the two diseases under the microscopic examination [9].

A good way to start is first identifying the two ideal or "pure" scenarios of both asthma and COPD, albeit they uncommonly exist in real world. Once the two diseases move toward each other, the "real" asthma and COPD patients begin to surface, and ACOS is nothing more but the overlap in between as summarized in Fig. 2.1.

2.1.2 Prevalence

Results of ACOS epidemiology studies vary because of multiple confounding factors including diverse ACOS definitions, tobacco-smoking population, age distribution, and study samples. In general population, the estimated prevalence of ACOS ranges from 1.6% to 4.5% based on studies in Italy, Latin America, and the United States [10–13]. ACOS prevalence among asthma population indicates a slightly higher percentage ranging from 13.3% to 61% in contrast with ACOS prevalence in COPD population, ranging from 12.1% to 55.2% [4, 10–23]. However, the lesser percentage of ACOS in COPD population could result from different COPD diagnostic criteria [24].

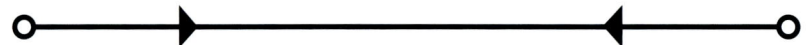

Characteristics	"Pure" Asthma	ACOS	"Pure" COPD
Usual Onset Age	<20-year-old	After early adulthood	>40-year-old
History	Personal and/or family history of atopy	Having history of either atopy or exposure to noxious particles and gases or both	History of exposure to tobacco smoking and/or biomass fuels
Respiratory Symptoms	"On or off" of intermittent symptoms with triggers	Persistent but highly varied symptoms	"Better or worse" of continuous symptoms not necessarily related to triggers
Lung Function	Variable airflow obstruction with reversibility	Persistent airflow obstruction with reversibility	Persistent or fixed airflow obstruction with low/no reversibility
Time Course	Symptoms do not worsen over time and more response to treatment	Slowly progressing symptoms over time and variable response to treatment	Symptoms progress over time and less response to treatment
Airway Inflammation	Eosinophilic	Eosinophilic and/or neutrophilic	Neutrophilic
Chest X-ray	Normal	From normal finding to hyperinflation	Hyperinflation and other changes of COPD

Fig. 2.1 Asthma, COPD, and ACOS in a longitudinal fashion with distinguished characteristics

2.1.3 Influence of Tobacco Smoking in Asthma

Similar to the public, active tobacco smoking in adult asthmatics ranges from 20% to 35% [25]. Clearly, tobacco smoking worsens asthma and parental smoking causes asthma exacerbation and possibly asthma development in children, but the evidence remains inconclusive to support tobacco smoking leading to adulthood asthma [26–30]. There is also lack of specific guidelines to treat cigarette-smoking asthmatics because early asthma researches excluded active smokers or past smokers with a 10 pack-year history [31, 32]. Nonetheless, tobacco smoking is associated with poor asthma control, worsening symptoms, and less responsive to glucocorticosteroids (GC) [33, 34]. While pulmonary growth matures in adolescent age and continues to decline thereafter, cigarette smokers with asthma have demonstrated an accelerated lung function reduction, fixed airway obstruction, and mostly neutrophilic inflammation which can result in COPD [35]. Importantly, studies have shown that the oxidative stress from tobacco smoking directly impacts on histone deacetylase-2 activity and causes GC insensitivity [36, 37]. This finding highlights the need for further research to help to restore GC sensitivity in asthmatic patients with tobacco smoking and ACOS and COPD patients [38].

2.1.4 Management and Future of ACOS

The earliest idea of ACOS can be traced back to 1961, and Orie and colleagues hypothesize that various forms of obstructive airway disease including asthma, chronic bronchitis, and emphysema should all be considered as a single common origin with different phenotypes/endotypes. They named the disease as "chronic nonspecific lung disease" [39]. Later, Fletcher and Pride proposed "Dutch hypothesis" that asthma and COPD are from the same source, supporting the concept of Orie, whereas Kraft and Barnes suggested that asthma and COPD are distinctly different, known as "British hypothesis" [39]. Recent data suggest

that there is no common genetic linkage between asthma and COPD, arguing against the "Dutch hypothesis" [18, 40]. Indeed, the term ACOS merely represents the late return of the longstanding conception between the two most common obstructive airway diseases. Since the absence of a clear definition and clinical trials of ACOS, the complexities of ACOS appear to be apparent, and ACOS research remains at a very preliminary stage.

However, the fact that ACOS has not turned out to be simple and unchallenging does not reduce the value of ACOS. When it is correctly diagnosed and managed, it is a very powerful guidance for the precision care of severe asthmatics. It has been recognized that COPD patients with eosinophilic or Th2 high type respond better to GC and vice versa, while asthma with neutrophilic or Th2 low type does not respond to GC well [41, 42]. Correctly differentiating asthma between Th2 high and low subgroup is the key to diagnosis and treatment of ACOS [43]. The differences in pathophysiology and treatment between type 2 high and low asthma will be further discussed elsewhere in this book.

Many authors advocate to abandoning the term ACOS. The actual underlying reason is that they felt no need to create a new vague term on the top of the already blurred definition of asthma or COPD [44, 45]. The definitions of asthma and COPD have become vague in order to try to cover their own overlaps, but many physicians get confused whether to call the subgroup of patients "asthma" or "COPD," thus the advent of ACOS. ACOS, the oversimplified terminology, has to be considered on a longitudinal line that contains clear directions coming from either "pure" asthma (eosinophilic) or "pure" COPD (neutrophilic) and moves toward to each other, as depicted in Fig. 2.1. Alternatively, the other way is to discard the current concept of asthma, COPD, and ACOS and put them all under an umbrella of the proposed term, "inflammatory lung disease," which is comprised of "eosinophilic," "neutrophilic," and "paucigranulocytic" types. Figure 2.2 summarizes treatment approaches depending on the inflammatory sub-

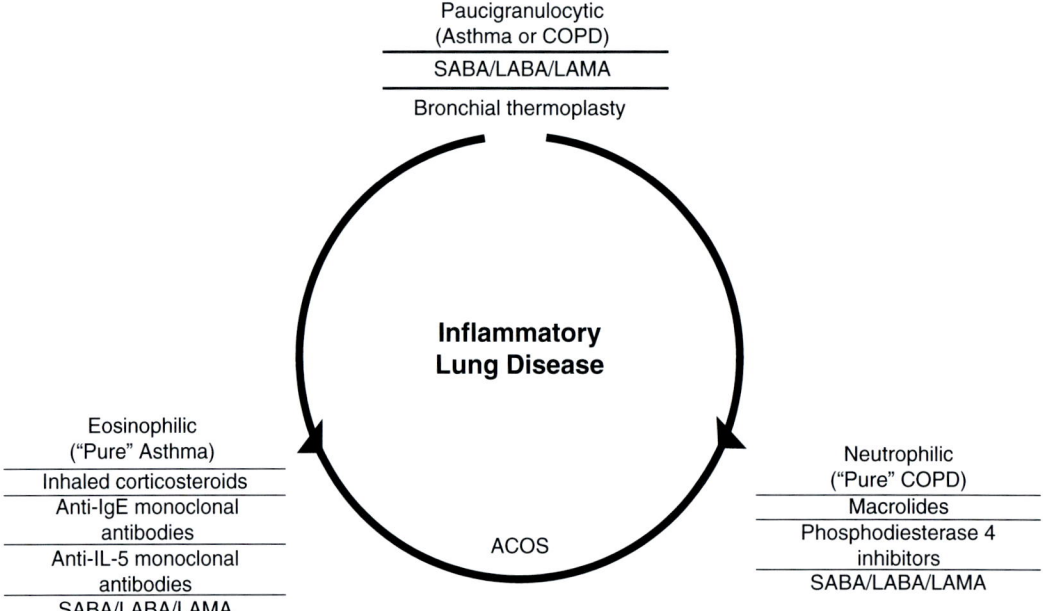

Fig. 2.2 Concept of "inflammatory lung disease," its different subtypes, and current treatments

groups. Future studies are required to fill this important gap between asthma and COPD, as they will help to precisely diagnose and manage this subgroup of asthma patients.

2.2 Comorbid Conditions of Severe Asthma

Although asthma could not be cured, control of asthma can be achieved in the majority of patients with combinations of appropriate medications, education, and environmental control [6, 46]. While experts have considered asthma as a treatable chronic disease, worldwide data including emergency department visits, the frequency of hospitalizations, and quality of life have shown that asthma remains to be improved in terms of its diagnosis and management [47]. There are several explanations to explain this enigma: (1) different phenotypes/endotypes that are all accommodated in this heterogeneous "asthma" category; (2) undertreatment due to either difficulty with inhalational device administration, lack of education, or poor adherence to medications; (3) misdiagnosis of asthma with it mimicking other disease such as vocal cord dysfunction (VCD); and (4) uncontrollable known, unknown, avoidable, and unavoidable allergens and irritants in the environment. Yet, another essential but often overlooked aspect leading to severe or recalcitrant asthma is the comorbid conditions. Some or all symptoms assessed for asthma could be contributed from either comorbid or coexisting condition [1, 6, 48]. Failure to identify and treat comorbid conditions in asthma is common.

The term "comorbid condition" used in this chapter refers to the diseases that participate in the pathophysiology of asthma and its acute exacerbation and coexist without necessary contribution to asthma. It is sometimes difficult to differentiate asthma and comorbid conditions, but both need to be diagnosed and treated properly. Like any other chronic diseases, asthma, particularly severe asthma with complex comorbid conditions, requires entire individual assessment, starting from a comprehensive and detailed medical history and physical examination.

In the present chapter, the main comorbid conditions associated with asthma and its acute exacerbation are reviewed in detail and summarized in Table 2.1.

Table 2.1 Testing and treatment of asthma comorbid conditions

Comorbidity	Diagnostic approach	Treatment
Respiratory infections (virus, bacteria, fungus)	Serology testing and culture *Aspergillus* skin prick and serology testing	Specific treatment to culprit pathogens Corticosteroids if allergic reaction (ABPA)
Rhinitis and rhinosinusitis	Skin prick and serum-specific IgE testing Rhinolaryngoscopy Sinus radiography/CT scan	Allergen avoidance Allergen immunotherapy Antihistamines and corticosteroids (oral and intranasal) Nasal saline irrigation Leukotriene receptor antagonists Antibiotics when relevant Surgery
Gastroesophageal reflux disease	Rhinolaryngoscopy/ esophagogastroduodenoscopy Manometry 24-h PH probe testing Intraluminal impedance testing Upper GI series	Lifestyle modification Antacid therapy (including proton pump inhibitor, H2 blocker) Surgical intervention
Obesity	BMI and other obesity measurements	Weight loss (including diet, exercise, medical and surgical treatment)
Obstructive sleep apnea	Polysomnography (portable or laboratory)	Weight loss Continuous positive airway pressure and other second line treatment
Psychopathologies	Psychological evaluation	Psychotherapy Psychiatrist referral
Vocal cord dysfunction	Laryngoscopy with or without challenge	Speech therapy and psychotherapy Breathing training

2.2.1 Respiratory Infections

The airways are continuously exposed to different irritants, allergens, and microorganisms such as bacteria, virus, and fungus. Respiratory infections can be easily transmitted between upper and lower airways due to similarities in their mucosal structures and innate and adaptive immune cascades [49]. In asthmatics, both innate and adaptive immune responses may be impaired [50]. Among diverse pathogens, viruses are particularly recognized as a common cause and accounted as high as 80–85% of pediatric and 80% of adult asthma exacerbations [51, 52]. Rhinoviruses are the most frequently detected virus in both pediatric and adult asthmatics [53]. Other well-known viruses involved in asthma exacerbation are respiratory syncytial viruses in infants and influenza viruses in adults [53]. The increased viral load in asthmatic subjects by decreased Th1 responses and augmented Th2 responses can lead to airway inflammation and asthma exacerbations [54]. This finding is also reinforced by eliminating seasonal peaks in virus-induced asthma exacerbations with the administration of omalizumab, which is an anti-IgE antibody used to control the Th2 responses [55].

Other atypical bacteria such as *Mycoplasma pneumoniae* and *Chlamydia pneumoniae* have been implicated in asthma exacerbations and also a long-term decline in lung function [56]. Regarding fungi, allergic bronchopulmonary aspergillosis is typically associated with asthma and can masquerade as severe asthma (discussed later in this chapter) [57]. Yet, the exact effect of atypical bacterial and fungi exposure on asthma morbidity requires further studies to explore.

2.2.2 Rhinitis and Rhinosinusitis

Approximately 20–50% of subjects with allergic rhinitis have asthma, whereas more than 80% asthma subjects have rhinitis [58–61]. Atopy is not an isolated linkage between asthma and rhinitis because evidence reveals the similar association of asthma with both allergic and nonallergic rhinitis [62]. Although the "united airways" concept is a somewhat arbitrary slogan, it does suggest that upper and lower airway inflammation are related each other [63, 64]. Research has demonstrated that segmental bronchial allergen provocation in nonasthmatic allergic rhinitis subjects induces nasal allergic inflammation, while nasal allergen provocation in allergic rhinitis subjects results in generalized airway inflammation [65, 66].

Chronic rhinosinusitis (CRS), another common upper airway inflammatory disease, accounts for up to 75% of asthmatic patients, irrespective of asthma severity, although the more extensive CRS is associated with more severe and refractory asthma [67]. CRS with nasal polyps is characterized by eosinophilic Th2-skewed inflammation, driven by interleukin (IL)-5 and eotaxin, which induces eosinophil chemotaxis, activation, and survival [68]. Further studies have demonstrated the presence of specific IgE to *Staphylococcus aureus* enterotoxin (*Staphylococcus aureus* colonization is a Th2-modifying and Th2-aggravating factor in CRS), high IL-5, and increased total IgE concentration within the nasal polyps as a predictor of concomitant asthma [69, 70]. A subcategory of nasal polyps, aspirin-exacerbated respiratory disease (AERD), is associated with aspirin sensitization and another severe asthma phenotype (discussed later in this chapter) [71].

2.2.3 Gastroesophageal Reflux Disease (GERD)

Numerous studies have determined the close connection between GERD and asthma. On average, 70% of adult asthma patients report to have GERD symptom(s) [72–74], and 67% of adult [75–81] and 56% of pediatric [82–89] asthmatics have abnormal esophageal pH testing. There is no definite cause-and-effect relationship other than vicious cycle between asthma and GERD. Asthma can promote GERD via changes in intrathoracic pressure and asthma medications alter esophageal sphincter pressure [90].

Conversely, GERD can provoke asthma through neurogenic reflexes and induce aspiration-triggered inflammation [90]. GERD could also lead to laryngopharyngeal hypersensitivity and hyperreactivity, which often result in VCD-mimicking asthma.

Despite the strong correlation between asthma and GERD, there is inconsistent data whether or not the effective treatment of GERD improves asthma outcome. A Cochrane review in 2003 has demonstrated no overall improvement including asthma symptoms, medications, and lung function in asthmatic subjects with GERD following anti-reflux treatment although subgroups of patients may gain benefit [91]. Subsequently, multiple studies also have failed to demonstrate asthma outcome improvement aiming for asymptomatic GERD and proximal esophageal reflux patients [92, 93]. Results from other clinical trials favoring asthma outcome are seen but reserved for moderate to severe GERD patients who require surgical intervention [94–96]. In short, only a subgroup of asthma patients benefits from treating GERD, and the decision to treat GERD has to be individualized, remembering long-term proton pump inhibitor therapy is not as benign as thought [97–99].

2.2.4 Obesity and Obstructive Sleep Apnea (OSA)

Obesity has been increasing worldwide and associated with growing asthma prevalence [90]. Several prospective studies and meta-analyses have shown higher adiposity or BMI as early as infancy can be a risk of asthma development [100–103]. In addition, multiple researches and a systemic review assessing the effect of weight reduction in obesity have demonstrated an improvement in asthma symptoms, medication burden, and overall asthma control [104–107]. Obesity-related asthma appears to be a distinct phenotype characterized by low eosinophilic inflammation, low-resting lung volumes, and less response to conventional asthma medications, particularly to ICS [108–111]. Such unresponsiveness to ICS is still elusive [111]. Furthermore, obese patients who make urgent visits for respiratory symptoms are more likely to be misdiagnosed as asthma [112]. Finally, apart from asthma, obesity itself has an association with a wide range of other comorbid conditions including GERD and OSA, which may compound the underlying respiratory disease [108]. To achieve the best outcome, it is critical to determine the dominant composition of obesity whether or not a patient has an obesity-related phenotype of asthma, obesity misdiagnosed as asthma, or asthma with comorbid obesity.

As OSA is often tied to obesity and weight loss improves both conditions, the actual relationship between asthma and OSA is obscured [113, 114]. Nevertheless, both the mechanical changes in OSA and the pro-inflammatory triggers from oxidative stress can affect the airways [115]. The usage of chronic and/or frequent bursts of systemic GC for asthma can impact substantially on the development of OSA or exacerbate the underlying OSA [113]. Judicious usage of systemic GC is important to prevent OSA, and continuous positive airway pressure is essential to treat OSA and subsequently help asthma [116–118].

2.2.5 Psychopathologies and Breathing Dysfunction

While schizophrenia, bipolar, and personality disorders do not correlate with asthma patients, general psychological disorders such as depression, anxiety, and panic disorders in asthmatics are more frequent than the general population [48, 119–124]. Patients with severe or refractory asthma often express more anxious, frustrated feeling and even lack of trust to physicians. These psychological conditions not only cause inadequate symptom detection and perception but impair medication compliance and even follow-up adherence [123–127]. Increased urgent care visits and hospitalization are reported in asthmatics with these psychological conditions [128, 129]. Psychological interventions in pediatric asthma patients have been reviewed in several analyses but lack substantial evidence to be conclusive [130–133]. Based on the positive results from specialists treating well-defined psychopathologies, appropriate psychological interventions should be offered to selected asthma patients [134].

There are a few breathing dysfunction conditions that can mimic asthma, and they are associated with psychopathologies [135]. Hyperventilation syndrome can affect up to 10% of the population and more prevalent in female asthmatics [136]. Successful respiratory physiotherapy targeting this over-breathing status has been noted [137]. Other breathing dysfunction conditions can come from either supraglottic or glottic dysfunction. VCD is defined as a paradoxical adduction of the vocal cords during inspiration and can be concomitant in up to 50% asthma patients [138]. Specific questionnaire and rhinoscopy have been developed to help identify this condition, and both speech therapy and/or psychotherapy have shown effective in treating VCD [139–141].

2.3 Allergic Bronchopulmonary Aspergillosis and Severe Asthma

Allergic bronchopulmonary aspergillosis (ABPA) is a progressive lung disease caused by airway hypersensitivity to fungi, mostly *Aspergillus fumigatus* (A*f*). Atopic individuals are linked to ABPA. The inflammatory response in favor of Th2 over Th1 leads to activation of IL-4, IL-5, and IL-13, and IgE synthesis and eosinophil chemotaxis. ABPA has been associated in patients with asthma and cystic fibrosis and less frequent with other diseases like the chronic granulomatous disease. ABPA is mostly caused by A*f* and less commonly with other fungi such as *Candida* species named as allergic bronchopulmonary mycosis.

Physicians should suspect and include APBA in the differential diagnosis in severe asthmatics with elevated total IgE and eosinophil level in serum or sputum, pulmonary infiltrates, and bronchiectasis [142]. While mostly largely the diagnosis of ABPA can be made with typical features and matched with the criteria, some patients may have an absence of these findings which mystify the diagnosis.

Complications of ABPA include copious sputum production, recurrent pneumonia, bronchiectasis, and loss of lung function. Early detection and diagnosis of ABPA will prevent lung damage or fibrosis. Treatment of ABPA is long-term GC and antifungal agents.

2.3.1 Prevalence

The exact prevalence of ABPA globally is undetermined. This is due to multiple factors such as lack of accepted diagnostic criteria, variability in the laboratory investigations, and under-recognition by physicians. As per the World Health Organization, out of the 193 million asthmatic patients worldwide, 4,837,000 patients are diagnosed with ABPA [143]. Other reports demonstrate that it affects 1–2% of asthmatic patients, 25–28% of asthmatics with a positive skin test to *Aspergillus*, 7–14% in GC-dependent asthmatics, and 2–15% of patients with cystic fibrosis [144–146].

2.3.2 Historical Preview

In 1952, Hinson et al. first reported ABPA in three patients with multiple manifestations including recurrent episodes of wheezing, elevated serum eosinophils count, chronic sputum production, fever, chest x-rays infiltrations, and evidence of *Aspergillus* in histological methods [147]. In 1968, Patterson et al. identified the first case of ABPA in the United States [148]. In 1897, Renon was the first to associate asthma and aspergillosis. In 1987, Greenberger and Patterson suggested a diagnostic criterion, which was refined by Schwartz and Greenberger in 1991 [149].

2.3.3 *Aspergillus* and Relationship with Asthma

ABPA is a result of hypersensitivity reaction of A*f* in the airways. The size of airborne *Aspergillus* spore is 2–3 μm, meaning it can reach the alveoli through inhalation. The spores then germinate in the inflamed airway, and the hyphae can be found in the mucus of the bronchi. The spores can grow at temperatures from 15 °C (59 °F) to 53 °C (127.4 °F). Asthma patients can have exacerbations when exposed to the mold-rich environment. A*f* is found in air samples from both indoor and water-damaged walls or ceilings.

In 2005, Maurya V et al. further investigated the relationship between sensitization to *Aspergillus* and occurrence of APBA in patients with asthma. A total of 105 asthmatic patients were involved in the study. The subjects underwent skin testing for *Aspergillus* and serum antigens of *Aspergillus*, and specific IgG against *Aspergillus* was measured. The results demonstrated an increase in the severity of asthma with *Aspergillus* sensitization. The authors concluded that ABPA should be excluded in all patients with *Aspergillus*-sensitive asthma [150]. The earlier study already confirmed the positive relationship between mold allergen exposure and severity of asthma in the study by Zureik M et al. [151]. 1132 patients aged 20–44 years with current asthma and their skin prick test results were investigated. Asthma severity was classified based on forced expiratory volume in one second (FEV1), the number of asthma attacks, hospital admissions for breathing problems, and the use of GC in the past 12 months. Results showed the increased frequency of sensitization to molds (*Alternaria alternata* or *Cladosporium herbarum*, or both) related with increasing asthma severity.

2.3.4 Pathophysiology

The pathogenesis of ABPA is not fully elucidated. Genetic factors are involved, including HLA antigens (DR2/DR5 and DR4/DR7), IL-10 and surfactant protein polymorphisms, and genetic mutations in cystic fibrosis transmembrane conductance regulator [152–155]. Patients with underlying airway disease, such as asthma, have a concomitantly increased mucus secretion and diminished mucociliary clearance. This leads to an increase in spore trapping with decreased clearance [150]. This animates germination of spores and release of antigenic proteins that aggravate the immune reactions. The *Aspergillus* allergens induce the immune response that involves IgE (type 1)- and IgG-mediated (type 3) reactions that further stimulate an intense inflammatory cascade in the airway than asthma alone. Further complications occur due to the dilatation in the proximal bronchi which is also filled with the mucus plus containing both eosinophils and fungal hyphae. This dilatation augments inflammatory reaction and eventually leads to bronchiectasis and airway obstruction [156].

Reactions to fungal allergens stimulate the humoral immune response mediated through the elevation in Af-specific IgG, IgA, and IgE [157]. Another form of response may occur in ABPA patients, and underlying asthma is the reaction after an acute exposure to already colonized Af in the bronchi, resulting in Th2- and IL-8-mediated response which leads to eosinophilic and neutrophilic inflammation, respectively. Histological findings in ABPA demonstrate eosinophilic pulmonary infiltrates, bronchocentric granulomatosis, mucoid impaction of bronchi, and bronchiectasis. Af allergen causes Th2 cell recruitment, which in turn releases IL-5, a cytokine that recruits eosinophils and B cells. The eosinophils then release their granular contents that promote an inflammatory response. The B cells promote immunoglobulin production. This is determined by serum elevation of Af-specific IgE and IgG, which are used for diagnostic purposes [155, 158]. The fungal proteases initiate the neutrophilic inflammatory response, which acts on epithelial cells and macrophages of the bronchi and causes the release of IL-8, recruiting neutrophils. Granular products of neutrophils further propagate the inflammatory response [155].

2.3.5 Clinical Features and Diagnosis

ABPA occurs in patients with uncontrolled asthma or cystic fibrosis. ABPA in severe asthmatics usually presents with worsening of respiratory symptoms such as frequent wheezing, increase in dyspnea, cough with thick, brownish sputum or plugs of mucus, and rarely hemoptysis [159]. Histologic features include eosinophilic debris and *Aspergillus* hyphae. Asthma plus systemic manifestation such as fever, weight loss, and fatigue should make physicians suspect ABPA. Typical radiologic findings, including central bronchiectasis, can be present in most ABPA patients. Other chest x-ray findings include pulmonary parenchymal infiltrates and fibrotic changes. A physician should be aware that ABPA comprises from mild to severe, and the latter may present with central bronchiectasis or end-stage lung fibrosis with respiratory failure. There are different criteria proposed for ABPA diagnosis with no accepted one unified criteria. Earlier reports for ABPA diagnosis involve asthma, serum eosinophilia, positive *Aspergillus* immediate skin test, and presence of precipitins to *Aspergillus* antigens [160].

Further classification involves the presence of central bronchiectasis or without bronchiectasis [161]. More specific assays for IgG to *Aspergillus* can be made due to the lack of specificity of *Aspergillus* precipitin assays [162]. As mentioned above, Greenberger and Patterson suggested a diagnostic criterion, which was refined by Schwartz and Greenberger in 1991 [149]. The obstacles for ABPA diagnostic criteria are due to the recent definition of severe asthma with fungal sensitization and patients with severe asthma plus coexistent fungal sensitization [163, 164].

The main differential diagnosis for ABPA-S is severe asthma with fungal sensitization, and the level of serum total IgE is considered the first distinguishing feature with a level higher than 1000 ng/mL in ABPA. Patients with levels between 500 and 1000 ng/mL should be closely monitored for development of ABPA with follow-up IgE level monitored every 6 weeks [165]. Stages of ABPA are illustrated in Table 2.2.

- *Diagnostic criteria for ABPA—central bronchiectasis* [166]
- For a diagnosis of ABPA-CB, there should be a minimum of five criteria:
  - Asthma
  - Proximal bronchiectasis (dilated bronchi in the inner two-thirds of the chest field on CT scan)
  - Immediate cutaneous reactivity to *Aspergillus* species

Table 2.2 Stages of ABPA

Stage	Acute	Remission	Exacerbation	Corticosteroid-dependent asthma	End-stage fibrosis
Symptoms	Fever, cough, chest pain, hemoptysis, sputum	No active complaint. Patient is off prednisolone >6 months	Relapse of acute symptoms	Persistent complaint of wheezing and cough despite using oral corticosteroid	Cyanosis or dyspnea
Imaging	Infiltrates of upper or middle lobes	Resolution of infiltrates	New infiltrates	Infiltrates maybe absent or only intermittent	Fibrotic, bullous, or cavitary lesions
Serum IgE	Elevated	Normal or slightly elevated	Elevated	Normal or elevated	Maybe normal

Adapted from Greenberger et al. [149]

- Elevated serum total IgE (>417 KU/L or 1000 ng/mL)
- Elevated serum A*f*-IgE and/or A*f*-IgG
- *Diagnostic criteria for ABPA—without bronchiectasis* [166]
  - Asthma.
  - Immediate cutaneous reactivity to *Aspergillus* species.
  - Elevated serum total IgE (>417 KU/L or 1000 ng/mL).
  - Elevated serum A*f*-IgE and/or A*f*-IgG.
  - Chest x-ray infiltrates may not be present. No bronchiectasis.

Most ABPA patients demonstrate immediate skin reactivity to A*f* [155, 167, 168]. Spirometry may show airflow obstruction, worsening vital capacity, and FEV1.

Evidence of *Aspergillus* sensitization is essential to make the diagnosis of ABPA, through either immediate skin test or serum *Aspergillus*-specific IgE. The lack of sensitivity to *Aspergillus* excludes ABPA except in the presence of other fungi causing airway disease. Both serum and skin testing are required to determine fungal sensitization [155]. Reactivity to the antigens Asp f 1, Asp f 3, Asp f 4, and Asp f 6 appears to be dominant in asthma patients. Antibodies against Asp 4 and Asp 6 have a higher sensitivity and specificity [169].

A threshold of 1000 IU/mL to make a diagnosis of ABPA was suggested by Agarwal [170]. Certain reports suggest a serum total IgE level of 1000 ng/mL for a suspicion of ABPA while rec-

ognizing that it is not the case in certain patients. Corticosteroids may lower the serum IgE levels. A 35% reduction in serum total IgE reflects the remission of ABPA, excluding serum total IgE levels of less than 2500 IU/mL [171].

Serum eosinophilia is another common finding in ABPA in addition to atopic diseases. ABPA patients may have sputum hyphae which indicate the presence of *Aspergillus*.

2.3.6 Radiologic Findings

Pulmonary opacities frequently manifest in ABPA. Involvement of the large airways may show transitory opacities, thickened airway walls and central bronchiectasis, mucus plugging, atelectasis, and significant pulmonary collapse. Opacification of the parenchymal lung in high-resolution computed tomography could be an initial finding in the early stage of the disease, with the tendency to progress to collapse or parenchymal scarring, often extending to the pleura [172]. A diagnostic finding in ABPA is central bronchiectasis with a predilection of the upper lobes. Bronchiectasis at lobar, segmental levels or involving the majority of airways is the characteristic finding in ABPA [173].

2.3.7 Histopathologic Findings

Diagnosis of ABPA does not require a pathological specimen, but a lung biopsy showing

Aspergillus colonization supports the diagnosis. Eosinophilic and lymphocytic infiltration in the airway is another common histological finding, and tissue sample may include other findings such as granulomas with distal exudative bronchiolitis, mucoid impaction, goblet cell hyperplasia, and fibrosis.

2.3.8 Treatment

The treatment goal is to relieve symptoms, prevent exacerbations, and stop the progression into central bronchiectasis and irreversible fibrosis.

2.3.8.1 Glucocorticosteroids (GCs)

The mainstay of treatment for ABPA is systemic GC. Serum total IgE should be monitored during treatment [161]. An example of systemic GC regime is prednisone 0.5 mg/kg daily for first 2 weeks followed by every other day for the next 3 months. A higher dose and longer duration, with the aim to prevent disease relapse, have been suggested. The absence of symptoms doesn't rule out active disease and serum total IgE level every 1–2 months to be used as a guide. If there's further serum total IgE elevation from baseline, GC dosage should be increased [174].

Acute exacerbations of ABPA should be managed with a higher dose of GC. A suggested dose of prednisone is 0.5–1.0 mg/kg/day for 1–2 weeks, followed by 0.5 mg/kg/day for 6–12 weeks on clinical remission. In case of life-threating situation, high dose of intravenous GC can be used [175]. GC should be tapered after symptom improvement. Other experts suggest using alternative-day GC regimen as an option. A combination of GC with itraconazole is proven successful in symptom improvement and a decline in total serum IgE. The antifungal treatment will be discussed in the following section.

GCs have become a crucial part in ABPA management. A patient may become steroid dependent, and physicians should monitor adverse events and interfere as soon as signs of side effects appear. If a decision is made to start long-term systemic GC, then vitamin D and calcium supplements should be prescribed.

2.3.8.2 Antifungal Agents

Antifungal therapy is adjunctive, and it has been associated with reduced airway inflammation and aimed to minimized airway damaged associated with bronchiectasis. Experts recommended a minimum 6-month period treatment in association with systemic corticosteroid.

Stevens et al. reported the effectiveness of itraconazole in a randomized, double-blind clinical trial in patients with GC-dependent ABPA. The participants received oral itraconazole 200 mg twice daily versus placebo for 16 weeks. Results showed decreased GC requirement in 46% of treatment group versus 19% in the placebo group [176]. Another study by Wark et al. is to assess the role of itraconazole, in a randomized, double-blind, placebo-controlled trial involving 29 patients with ABPA [177]. Fifteen patients received 400 mg of itraconazole daily versus 14 patients with placebo for 16 weeks. The results demonstrated a reduction in sputum eosinophils in the treatment group with no decrease in the placebo group. Wark et al. assessed the role of oral ketoconazole 400 mg/day for 12 months, and results showed symptom reduction and a decline in immunological marker [178]. Voriconazole is shown to be effective as an alternative antifungal in case series [179].

2.3.8.3 Biologics

Elevated IgE has been associated with ABPA patients, and the benefit of the anti-IgE antibody has been documented in severe asthmatics with decreased asthma exacerbation rates. Omalizumab, a monoclonal antibody to IgE, has been evaluated, and some studies have published its effect in ABPA patients. The role of omalizumab seems to be promising, with the reduction in asthma exacerbation and the dosage of the systemic GC.

A study by Tillie et al. to assess the role of omalizumab involving 16 patients with ABPA showed a reduction of exacerbations [180]. Further research will be needed for better understanding of the pathophysiology, appropriate dose, and treatment duration for omalizumab in ABPA.

2.4 Aspirin-Exacerbated Respiratory Disease and Severe Asthma

Aspirin-exacerbated respiratory disease (AERD) is a disease manifested by a triad of asthma, nasal polyposis, and aspirin sensitivity. Other nomenclature for this disease includes Samter's triad, aspirin triad, and aspirin-sensitivity triad, and it is also known as aspirin-intolerant asthma, aspirin (ASA)-sensitive asthma, Widal triad, Francis triad, or Fernand-Widal triad. Some authors consider this disease as a subclass of chronic rhinosinusitis, while others reported the association under a subset of patients with asthma. In general, it affects adult population and is infrequently diagnosed in pediatric patients. The pathological mechanism proposed in this disease involves alterations in arachidonate metabolism and the overproduction of cysteinyl leukotrienes (cysLTs); other proposed theories will be discussed below. Eosinophilic and mast cell inflammatory process has also been involved in AERD. This inflammatory process can be initiated even before starting aspirin.

2.4.1 Historical Preview

In 1902, Hirschberg was first to describe a hypersensitivity reaction to ASA, and this is followed by several descriptions of hypersensitivity reactions to nonsteroidal anti-inflammatory drugs (NSAIDs). In 1911, Gilbert G was first to recognize aspirin-induced asthmatic dyspnea [181]. Further reports followed by Widal MF et al. as a triad of symptoms consists of nasal polyposis in patients with nonallergic induced asthma and ASA sensitivity [182]. In 1967–1968, the triad was promoted further by Samter and Beers and became known as "Samter's triad" [183]. This relationship between asthma, nasal polyposis, and ASA sensitivity has been recognized and widespread after Samter's publication in 1968. The name Samter's triad or AERD has been widely used since then. Desensitization to ASA was first described by Zeiss and Lockey in 1976. Szczeklik and Stevenson developed ASA desensitization protocols in the 1980s. The pathophysiology of AERD was described by Szczeklik in 1990, based on the cyclooxygenase theory.

2.4.2 Prevalence and Presentations

The prevalence of AERD is variable, based on multiple factors such as the methods of diagnosis whether by drug challenge or history alone and age of presentation. Studies have shown not much correlation between AERD and atopy.

In a study of 300 patients with suspected AERD, Berges-Gimeno MP et al. reported a female predominance (57%) comparing to male (43%) with no difference between both genders regarding symptom severity [184]. In 2004, Jenkins C et al. used oral ASA challenge as a diagnostic tool and reported a 21% of asthmatic adults and 5% of asthmatic children's suffering from ASA sensitivity. In 2006, Pfaar O et al. reported the incidence of ASA hypersensitivity ranging from 0.6% to 2.5% in general population, while in adult asthmatics the range is higher 4.3–11% [185]. In 2015, Rajan JP et al. report a prevalence of AERD as 7% in typical adult asthmatic patients, and the number is doubled in severe asthmatics [186]. Hedman J et al. report the prevalence of ASA intolerance 5.7%, with only 1.2% experiencing aspirin-induced asthma. Szczeklik A et al. reported the mean age of presentation as 30 years old in a study of 500 aspirin-intolerant asthma patients [187]. Similarly, Berges-Gimeno MP et al. found the average age at the onset of AERD is 34 years old [184].

2.4.3 Diagnosis

Diagnosis of AERD can be challenging due to no currently available in vitro testing. Clinicians should consider AERD in patients with difficult-to-control asthma as a differential diagnosis. Patients should be asked for a history of previous naso-ocular symptoms, any respiratory reaction, or flare-up of asthma after ingestions of NSAIDs on at least two separate occasions. Exacerbations of respiratory symptoms can occur within a few minutes and up to 3 h after ingestion [187]. Once suspecting for AERD, ASA challenge is essential to confirm the diagnosis, which has been established and widely used.

AERD patients that react to ASA can also react to other NSAIDs, which is related to inhibition of the cyclooxygenase (COX)-1 enzyme and/or alteration in the pathway between prostaglandin and leukotriene.

Aspirin challenge can be performed through different routes most commonly with oral administration in the United States. There are four routes to deliver ASA including oral, bronchial, nasal, and intravenous. Some authors have suggested nasal challenge for AERD patients with isolated nasal symptoms [188]. If the nasal challenge is negative, then the patient should be evaluated with either oral or bronchial route if high suspicion for AERD.

In oral challenge, patients are given with an initial dose around 20–40 mg followed by gradual up-titration to the top dose 325 mg as long as no reaction. Lung function and symptoms are monitored after each dose. A positive challenge is if FEV1 drops significantly and/or naso-ocular symptoms develop. In Europe, lysine aspirin, a soluble solution of 900 mg of lysine aspirin (Sanofi, Paris, France) which is equivalent to 500 mg of ASA, is used in both bronchial and nasal challenges, but this technique is not approved by the Food and Drug Administration in the United States [189]. Other in vitro study measuring peripheral blood basophil activation by flow cytometric technique may provide future diagnostic values [190].

Some investigators evaluated another approach to diagnose ASA sensitivity. White A et al. performed intranasal ketorolac challenge in 29 patients with AERD [191]. The results showed that nasal ketorolac challenge has a sensitivity of 78% and a specificity of 64%. The authors conclude that this approach is safe and considered as an alternative method.

AERD diagnosis can be challenging if a patient has unstable asthma; in such case, oral ASA challenge is not recommended, and the patient should be treated first to stabilize asthma. Challenge can be performed once asthma is stable.

2.4.4 Pathogenesis

The exact mechanism of AERD is yet to be explained. The pathogenesis is proposed from the abnormal metabolism of arachidonic acid in the lipoxygenase (LO) and COX pathways, and the results of unbalanced proinflammatory and anti-inflammatory mediators.

ASA is known to block COX-mediated prostanoid production, shunting arachidonic acid to the alternative LO metabolic pathway resulting in a decrease of prostaglandins and an increase in leukotriene production [192]. CysLTs are bronchoconstrictors, and they urge mucus secretion and increase vascular permeability. Increase production of cysLTs after ASA challenge has been validated in multiple studies [193]. Prostaglandin E2 (PGE2), a prostanoid synthesized by the COX pathway, is known to suppress the production of cysLTs through slowing the 5-LO pathway and suppresses mast cell activation [194]. Sestini P et al. validated the role of bronchodilation ability of PGE2 in the lungs through inhalation tests before aspirin challenge. Other studies confirmed that patients with AERD have a deficiency in PGE2 when compared with aspirin-tolerant and healthy control subjects [195]. NSAIDs are known to block COX-1 activity, which leads to decrease PGE2 synthesis and promote cysLTs production. Another study demonstrated that AERD patients have upregulated 5-LO pathway and further increase in cysLT production [188]. Patients with AERD have upregulated leukotriene C4 (LTC4) which is made by LTC4 synthase [196]. Leukotriene E4 (LTE4) is a metabolite of LTC4. Urinary LTE4 levels have been used to monitor the endogenous synthesis of cysLTs because of its stability. AERD patients have higher basal levels of urinary LTE4 when compared with aspirin-tolerant asthmatics [197]. Overexpression of cysLT receptor 1 is demonstrated in nasal inflammatory leukocytes, as well as a downregulation of receptor expression after ASA desensitization [198].

2.4.5 Management and Medications

The goal of AERD management is to avoid COX-1 inhibitors. Once AERD is diagnosed, an avoidance medication list of ASA and NSAIDs should be provided. The safety of COX-2 inhibitors in AERD has been evaluated. Simon RA et al. reported that there is no cross-sensitivity between COX-1 inhibitors and highly selective COX-2 inhibitors [199]. In 2001, Szczeklik A et al. showed that patients with asthma could tolerate COX-2 inhibitors (rofecoxib) with no significant fall in FEV1 and no significant change in mean urinary LTE4 [200]. A meta-analysis by Morales DR et al. demonstrated the safety of COX-2 inhibitors in AERD patients [201]. Acetaminophen is a weak COX-1 inhibitor that can be acceptable up to a dose of 650 mg in patients with AERD but not at the higher dose of 1000 mg according to few studies [202].

The other approach is to block the leukotriene pathway. There are two forms of anti-LT therapy approved for asthma patients in the United States: zileuton and montelukast/zafirlukast. Zileuton is a 5-LO inhibitor, partially blocking arachidonic acid conversion into leukotriene A4. Dahlen et al. demonstrated the ability of zileuton in decreasing the number of asthma exacerbations, improve pulmonary function, improve a sense of smell, and decrease nonspecific bronchial hyperreactivity to histamine [203]. The second form of anti-leukotriene therapy includes montelukast (10 mg daily) and zafirlukast (20 mg daily). The pharmacological mechanism is related to the ability of

binding to cysLT receptor 1. A double-blind placebo-controlled trial in by Dahlen SE et al. demonstrated that montelukast decreases asthma symptoms and improves pulmonary function and asthma-specific quality of life [204].

Proper management of nasal polyps is also required in AERD with intranasal GC in addition to the selective use of systemic GC. The duration of systemic GC is variable and depends on patients' clinical response. Topical decongestants such as oxymetazoline are a useful therapy in refractory nasal congestion not responding to GC. Antibiotics can be helpful in case of suspected acute bacterial infection causing an asthma flare-up. Other potential medications include oral antihistamines and oral decongestants although no substantial evidence supports these drugs.

2.4.6 Aspirin Desensitization

ASA desensitization should be considered as an essential part of management in AERD patients who required aspirin or if the conventional therapy has been failed. ASA desensitization has been shown to be safe and well tolerated. A standard oral ASA desensitization protocol is depicted in Table 2.3. The severity of the lung function decline should be evaluated before ASA desensitization.

In 2003, Berges-Gimeno et al. evaluated the long-term treatment benefit of ASA desensitization for 6 months and then followed for 1–5 years among

Table 2.3 Oral ASA challenge/desensitization protocol

Time	8 AM	11 AM	2 PM	5 PM
Day 1	20–40 mg	40–60 mg	60–100 mg	Instruction and discharge
Day 2	100 mg	160 mg	325 mg	Instruction and discharge

Clinical and objective evaluation performed every 30 min and as needed. Provoking dose is repeated; symptoms are treated as indicated. Provoking dose is defined as any reaction in upper/lower respiratory system, cutaneous manifestation/skin rash, gastrointestinal symptoms
After the patient is completely stabilized, the provoking dose can be repeated on day 1 (if there is time). Otherwise, the patient should be sent home, and the provoking dose should be repeated the next morning. FEV1 and clinical assessment every hour or with any symptoms
If nasal, gastrointestinal, or cutaneous reactions occur on day 1, pretreat with histamine1 and histamine2 blocker for the remainder of the challenge sequence. Generally, patients are challenged/treated with increasing doses of ASA over (in our table, we used 3 h as set time interval). In case a positive reaction, then this dose will be repeated until no response occurs, and dose is increased until a maximum dose is reached and tolerated

172 AERD patients [205]. The results showed significant clinical benefits including a decline in sinus infection rate, improvement in the sense of smell, and ameliorated asthma symptoms. There was a sustained benefit after 1 year of desensitization in most patients. Overall GC usage such as intranasal, inhaled, and oral was significantly reduced.

Intranasal ketorolac combined with oral ASA desensitization is another alternative and safe modality [206]. On day 1, the patient receives four metered nasal sprays, with 30-min observation between doses, followed by two doses of 60 mg oral ASA with 90-min interval. The patient will be observed and monitored for any signs or symptoms of the reaction and lung function. On day 2, the patient will have 150 mg followed by 325 mg of oral ASA within 3-h interval. This approach may shorten the challenge duration and improve the safety profile compared with the standard oral ASA desensitization.

2.4.7 Surgery

In refractory AERD, the surgical approach is considered to be a treatment of choice. The benefit of using endoscopic sinus surgery (ESS) in AERD needs to be further illustrated. Nakamura H et al. evaluated 22 AERD patients that underwent sinus surgery [207]. Patients reported improvement from surgical intervention although no comparison group was involved to validate the surgery. In 2006, Loehrl et al. had 31 AERD patients undergo ESS [208]. Patients reported postoperative improvement in a 10-year follow-up period and a decrease in emergency department visits for AERD/asthma exacerbations. ESS should be done to minimize the nasal polyp burden before ASA desensitization for AERD with severe nasal polyposis.

Conclusions

In summary, the pathogenesis of AERD involves an imbalance between leukotrienes and prostaglandins, and management of AERD can be challenging. ASA desensitization is a safe and specialized procedure that will improve the disease outcome while developing

tolerability to ASA and other cross-reacting NSAIDs. However, the benefits of long-term ASA therapy should be weighed against the risks such as the development of the gastrointestinal ulcer or bleeding as proton pump inhibitors could protect only the upper gastrointestinal tract. Surgical intervention in combination medical therapy may be a better approach in severe and refractory AERD cases.

References

1. van Schayck CP, Levy ML, Chen JC, Isonaka S, Halbert RJ. Coordinated diagnostic approach for adult obstructive lung disease in primary care. Prim Care Respir J. 2004;13(4):218–21.
2. Zeki AA, Schivo M, Chan A, Albertson TE, Louie S. The asthma-COPD overlap syndrome: a common clinical problem in the elderly. J Allergy (Cairo). 2011;2011:861926.
3. Gibson PG, Simpson JL. The overlap syndrome of asthma and COPD: what are its features and how important is it? Thorax. 2009;64(8):728–35.
4. Kauppi P, Kupiainen H, Lindqvist A, Tammilehto L, Kilpeläinen M, Kinnula VL, et al. Overlap syndrome of asthma and COPD predicts low quality of life. J Asthma. 2011;48(3):279–85.
5. Global Initiative for Asthma. Diagnosis of diseases of chronic airflow limitation: asthma, COPD and Asthma-COPD Overlap Syndrome (ACOS). www.ginasthma.org/. Accessed 1 July 2014.
6. Global Initiative for Asthma. 2016 GINA report, global strategy for asthma management and prevention. www.ginasthma.org/.
7. Global Initiative for Chronic Obstructive Lung Disease. Global strategy for diagnosis, management, and prevention of COPD. 2016. www.goldcopd.org/.
8. Postma DS, Rabe KF. The asthma-COPD overlap syndrome. N Engl J Med. 2015;373(13):1241–9.
9. Bourdin A, Serre I, Flamme H, Vic P, Neveu D, Aubas P, et al. Can endobronchial biopsy analysis be recommended to discriminate between asthma and COPD in routine practice? Thorax. 2004;59(6):488–93.
10. Diaz-guzman E, Khosravi M, Mannino DM. Asthma, chronic obstructive pulmonary disease, and mortality in the U.S. population. COPD. 2011;8(6):400–7.
11. Menezes AM, Montes de Oca M, Pérez-Padilla R, Nadeau G, Wehrmeister FC, Lopez-Varela MV, et al. Increased risk of exacerbation and hospitalization in subjects with an overlap phenotype: COPD-asthma. Chest. 2014;145(2):297–304.
12. Pleasants RA, Ohar JA, Croft JB, Liu Y, Kraft M, Mannino DM, et al. Chronic obstructive pulmonary

disease and asthma-patient characteristics and health impairment. COPD. 2014;11(3):256–66.

13. de Marco R, Pesce G, Marcon A, Accordini S, Antonicelli L, Bugiani M, et al. The coexistence of asthma and chronic obstructive pulmonary disease (COPD): prevalence and risk factors in young, middle-aged and elderly people from the general population. PLoS One. 2013;8(5):e62985.

14. Lamprecht B, McBurnie MA, Vollmer WM, Gudmundsson G, Welte T, Nizankowska-Mogilnicka E, et al. COPD in never smokers: results from the population-based burden of obstructive lung disease study. Chest. 2011;139(4):752–63.

15. Andersén H, Lampela P, Nevanlinna A, Säynäjäkangas O, Keistinen T. High hospital burden in overlap syndrome of asthma and COPD. Clin Respir J. 2013;7(4):342–6.

16. Iwamoto H, Gao J, Koskela J, Kinnula V, Kobayashi H, Laitinen T, et al. Differences in plasma and sputum biomarkers between COPD and COPD-asthma overlap. Eur Respir J. 2014;43(2):421–9.

17. Izquierdo-Alonso JL, Rodriguez-Gonzálezmoro JM, de Lucas-Ramos P, Unzueta I, Ribera X, Antón E, et al. Prevalence and characteristics of three clinical phenotypes of chronic obstructive pulmonary disease (COPD). Respir Med. 2013;107(5):724–31.

18. Hardin M, Cho M, McDonald ML, Beaty T, Ramsdell J, Bhatt S, et al. The clinical and genetic features of COPD-asthma overlap syndrome. Eur Respir J. 2014;44(2):341–50.

19. Hardin M, Silverman EK, Barr RG, Hansel NN, Schroeder JD, Make BJ, et al. The clinical features of the overlap between COPD and asthma. Respir Res. 2011;12:127.

20. Kitaguchi Y, Komatsu Y, Fujimoto K, Hanaoka M, Kubo K. Sputum eosinophilia can predict responsiveness to inhaled corticosteroid treatment in patients with overlap syndrome of COPD and asthma. Int J Chron Obstruct Pulmon Dis. 2012;7:283–9.

21. Wurst KE, Shukla A, Muellerova H, Davis KJ. Respiratory pharmacotherapy use in patients newly diagnosed with chronic obstructive pulmonary disease in a primary care setting in the UK: a retrospective cohort study. COPD. 2014;11(5):521–30.

22. Rhee CK, Yoon HK, Yoo KH, Kim YS, Lee SW, Park YB, et al. Medical utilization and cost in patients with overlap syndrome of chronic obstructive pulmonary disease and asthma. COPD. 2014;11(2):163–70.

23. Marsh SE, Travers J, Weatherall M, Williams MV, Aldington S, Shirtcliffe PM, et al. Proportional classifications of COPD phenotypes. Thorax. 2008;63(9):761–7.

24. Chang J, Mosenifar Z. Differentiating COPD from asthma in clinical practice. J Intensive Care Med. 2007;22(5):300–9.

25. Thomson NC, Chaudhuri R. Asthma in smokers: challenges and opportunities. Curr Opin Pulm Med. 2009;15(1):39–45.

26. Polosa R, Thomson NC. Smoking and asthma: dangerous liaisons. Eur Respir J. 2013;41(3):716–26.

27. Baena-cagnani CE, Gómez RM, Baena-cagnani R, Canonica GW. Impact of environmental tobacco smoke and active tobacco smoking on the development and outcomes of asthma and rhinitis. Curr Opin Allergy Clin Immunol. 2009;9(2):136–40.

28. Gilliland FD, Islam T, Berhane K, Gauderman WJ, McConnell R, Avol E, et al. Regular smoking and asthma incidence in adolescents. Am J Respir Crit Care Med. 2006;174(10):1094–100.

29. Coogan PF, Castro-webb N, Yu J, O'connor GT, Palmer JR, Rosenberg L. Active and passive smoking and the incidence of asthma in the Black Women's Health Study. Am J Respir Crit Care Med. 2015;191(2):168–76.

30. US Department of Health and Human Services. The health consequences of smoking: 50 years of progress. A report of the Surgeon General. Atlanta, GA: U.S. Department of Health and Human Services, Centers for Disease Control and Prevention, National Center for Chronic Disease Prevention and Health Promotion, Office on Smoking and Health; 2014.

31. Thomson NC, Spears M. Asthma guidelines and smokers: it's time to be inclusive. Chest. 2012;141(2):286–8.

32. Price D, Bjermer L, Popov TA, Chisholm A. Integrating evidence for managing asthma in patients who smoke. Allergy Asthma Immunol Res. 2014;6(2):114–20.

33. Thomson NC, Chaudhuri R, Heaney LG, Bucknall C, Niven RM, Brightling CE, et al. Clinical outcomes and inflammatory biomarkers in current smokers and exsmokers with severe asthma. J Allergy Clin Immunol. 2013;131(4):1008–16.

34. Bakakos P, Kostikas K, Loukides S. Smoking asthma phenotype: diagnostic and management challenges. Curr Opin Pulm Med. 2016;22(1):53–8.

35. Tamimi A, Serdarevic D, Hanania NA. The effects of cigarette smoke on airway inflammation in asthma and COPD: therapeutic implications. Respir Med. 2012;106(3):319–28.

36. Barnes PJ. Reduced histone deacetylase in COPD: clinical implications. Chest. 2006;129(1):151–5.

37. Kobayashi Y, Bossley C, Gupta A, Akashi K, Tsartsali L, Mercado N, et al. Passive smoking impairs histone deacetylase-2 in children with severe asthma. Chest. 2014;145(2):305–12.

38. Marwick JA, Adcock IM, Chung KF. Overcoming reduced glucocorticoid sensitivity in airway disease: molecular mechanisms and therapeutic approaches. Drugs. 2010;70(8):929–48.

39. Gelb AF, Nadel JA. Understanding the pathophysiology of the asthma-chronic obstructive pulmonary disease overlap syndrome. J Allergy Clin Immunol. 2015;136(3):553–5.

40. Smolonska J, Koppelman GH, Wijmenga C, Vonk JM, Zanen P, Bruinenberg M, et al. Common genes

underlying asthma and COPD? Genome-wide analysis on the Dutch hypothesis. Eur Respir J. 2014;44(4):860–72.

41. Tho NV, Park HY, Nakano Y. Asthma-COPD overlap syndrome (ACOS): a diagnostic challenge. Respirology. 2016;21(3):410–8.

42. Green RH, Brightling CE, Woltmann G, Parker D, Wardlaw AJ, Pavord ID. Analysis of induced sputum in adults with asthma: identification of subgroup with isolated sputum neutrophilia and poor response to inhaled corticosteroids. Thorax. 2002;57(10):875–9.

43. Wenzel SE. Asthma phenotypes: the evolution from clinical to molecular approaches. Nat Med. 2012;18(5):716–25.

44. Kostikas K, Clemens A, Patalano F. The asthma-COPD overlap syndrome: do we really need another syndrome in the already complex matrix of airway disease? Int J Chron Obstruct Pulmon Dis. 2016;11:1297–306.

45. Cazzola M, Rogliani P. Do we really need asthma-chronic obstructive pulmonary disease overlap syndrome? J Allergy Clin Immunol. 2016;138(4):977–83.

46. Boulet LP. Influence of comorbid conditions on asthma. Eur Respir J. 2009;33(4):897–906.

47. Peters SP, Ferguson G, Deniz Y, Reisner C. Uncontrolled asthma: a review of the prevalence, disease burden and options for treatment. Respir Med. 2006;100(7):1139–51.

48. Chanez P, Wenzel SE, Anderson GP, Anto JM, Bel EH, Boulet LP, et al. Severe asthma in adults: what are the important questions? J Allergy Clin Immunol. 2007;119(6):1337–48.

49. Baraniuk JN, Blaiss MS, Pattanaik D. Nonallergic rhinopathies and lower airway syndromes. In: Lockey RF, Ledford DK, editors. Asthma: comorbidities, coexisting conditions, & differential diagnosis. Oxford, NY: Oxford University Press; 2014. p. 244–59.

50. Mallia P, Johnston SL. How viral infections cause exacerbation of airway diseases. Chest. 2006;130(4):1203–10.

51. Johnston SL, Pattemore PK, Sanderson G, Smith S, Lampe F, Josephs L, et al. Community study of role of viral infections in exacerbations of asthma in 9-11 year old children. BMJ. 1995;310(6989):1225–9.

52. Nicholson KG, Kent J, Ireland DC. Respiratory viruses and exacerbations of asthma in adults. BMJ. 1993;307(6910):982–6.

53. Papadopoulos NG, Christodoulou I, Rohde G, Agache I, Almqvist C, Bruno A, et al. Viruses and bacteria in acute asthma exacerbations—a GA² LEN-DARE systematic review. Allergy. 2011;66(4):458–68.

54. Message SD, Laza-Stanca V, Mallia P, Parker HL, Zhu J, Kebadze T, et al. Rhinovirus-induced lower respiratory illness is increased in asthma and related to virus load and Th1/2 cytokine and IL-10 production. Proc Natl Acad Sci U S A. 2008;105(36):13562–7.

55. Busse WW, Morgan WJ, Gergen PJ, Mitchell HE, Gern JE, Liu AH, et al. Randomized trial of omalizumab (anti-IgE) for asthma in inner-city children. N Engl J Med. 2011;364(11):1005–15.

56. Sutherland ER, Martin RJ. Asthma and atypical bacterial infection. Chest. 2007;132(6):1962–6.

57. Denning DW, O'driscoll BR, Hogaboam CM, Bowyer P, Niven RM. The link between fungi and severe asthma: a summary of the evidence. Eur Respir J. 2006;27(3):615–26.

58. Bousquet J, Van Cauwenberge P, Khaltaev N. Allergic rhinitis and its impact on asthma. J Allergy Clin Immunol. 2001;108(5 Suppl):S147–334.

59. Demoly P, Bousquet J. The relation between asthma and allergic rhinitis. Lancet. 2006;368(9537):711–3.

60. Peters S. The impact of comorbid atopic disease on asthma: clinical expression and treatment. J Asthma. 2007;44(3):149–61.

61. Bousquet J, Khaltaev N, Cruz AA, Denburg J, Fokkens WJ, Togias A, et al. Allergic rhinitis and its impact on asthma (ARIA) 2008 update (in collaboration with the World Health Organization, GA(2)LEN and AllerGen). Allergy. 2008;63(Suppl 86):8–160.

62. Chawes BL, Bønnelykke K, Kreiner-møller E, Bisgaard H. Children with allergic and nonallergic rhinitis have a similar risk of asthma. J Allergy Clin Immunol. 2010;126(3):567–73.e1-8.

63. Rowe-jones JM. The link between the nose and lung, perennial rhinitis and asthma—is it the same disease? Allergy. 1997;52(36 Suppl):20–8.

64. Togias A. Mechanisms of nose-lung interaction. Allergy. 1999;54(Suppl 57):94–105.

65. Braunstahl GJ, Kleinjan A, Overbeek SE, Prins JB, Hoogsteden HC, Fokkens WJ. Segmental bronchial provocation induces nasal inflammation in allergic rhinitis patients. Am J Respir Crit Care Med. 2000;161(6):2051–7.

66. Braunstahl GJ, Overbeek SE, Kleinjan A, Prins JB, Hoogsteden HC, Fokkens WJ. Nasal allergen provocation induces adhesion molecule expression and tissue eosinophilia in upper and lower airways. J Allergy Clin Immunol. 2001;107(3):469–76.

67. Bresciani M, Paradis L, Des Roches A, Vernhet H, Vachier I, Godard P, et al. Rhinosinusitis in severe asthma. J Allergy Clin Immunol. 2001;107(1):73–80.

68. Otto BA, Wenzel SE. The role of cytokines in chronic rhinosinusitis with nasal polyps. Curr Opin Otolaryngol Head Neck Surg. 2008;16(3):270–4.

69. Bachert C, Zhang N, Holtappels G, De Lobel L, van Cauwenberge P, Liu S, et al. Presence of IL-5 protein and IgE antibodies to staphylococcal enterotoxins in nasal polyps is associated with comorbid asthma. J Allergy Clin Immunol. 2010;126(5):962–8. 968. e1-6

70. Kowalski ML, Cieślak M, Pérez-novo CA, Makowska JS, Bachert C. Clinical and immunologi-

cal determinants of severe/refractory asthma (SRA): association with staphylococcal superantigen-specific IgE antibodies. Allergy. 2011;66(1):32–8.

71. Ceylan E, Gencer M, San I. Nasal polyps and the severity of asthma. Respirology. 2007;12(2):272–6.

72. Perrin-Fayolle M, Bel A, Kofman J, Harf R, Montagnon B, Pacheco Y, et al. Asthma and gastro-esophageal reflux. Results of a survey over 150 cases (author's transl). Poumon Coeur. 1980;36(4):225–30.

73. Field SK, Underwood M, Brant R, Cowie RL. Prevalence of gastroesophageal reflux symptoms in asthma. Chest. 1996;109(2):316–22.

74. Sontag SJ, O'connell S, Miller TQ, Bernsen M, Seidel J. Asthmatics have more nocturnal gasping and reflux symptoms than nonasthmatics, and they are related to bedtime eating. Am J Gastroenterol. 2004;99(5):789–96.

75. Ducoloné A, Vandevenne A, Jouin H, Grob JC, Coumaros D, Meyer C, et al. Gastroesophageal reflux in patients with asthma and chronic bronchitis. Am Rev Respir Dis. 1987;135(2):327–32.

76. Nagel RA, Brown P, Perks WH, Wilson RS, Kerr GD. Ambulatory pH monitoring of gastro-oesophageal reflux in "morning dipper" asthmatics. BMJ. 1988;297(6660):1371–3.

77. Giudicelli R, Dupin B, Surpas P, Badier M, Charpin D, Lapicque JC, et al. Gastro-oesophagal reflux and respiratory manifestations: diagnostic approach, therapeutic indications and results. Ann Chir. 1990;44:552–4.

78. Sontag SJ, O'Connell S, Khandelwal S, Miller T, Nemchausky B, Schnell TG, et al. Most asthmatics have gastroesophageal reflux with or without bronchodilator therapy. Gastroenterology. 1990;99(3):613–20.

79. Demeester TR, Bonavina L, Iascone C, Courtney JV, Skinner DB. Chronic respiratory symptoms and occult gastroesophageal reflux. A prospective clinical study and results of surgical therapy. Ann Surg. 1990;211(3):337–45.

80. Larrain A, Carrasco E, Galleguillos F, Sepulveda R, Pope CE. Medical and surgical treatment of non-allergic asthma associated with gastroesophageal reflux. Chest. 1991;99(6):1330–5.

81. Kiljander TO, Salomaa ER, Hietanen EK, Terho EO. Gastroesophageal reflux in asthmatics: a double-blind, placebo-controlled crossover study with omeprazole. Chest. 1999;116(5):1257–64.

82. Friedland GW, Yamate M, Marinkovich VA. Hiatal hernia and chronic unremitting asthma. Pediatr Radiol. 1973;1(3):156–60.

83. Berquist WE, Rachelefsky GS, Kadden M, Siegel SC, Katz RM, Fonkalsrud E, et al. Gastroesophageal reflux-associated recurrent pneumonia and chronic asthma in children. Pediatrics. 1981;68(1):29–35.

84. Shapiro GG, Christie DL. Gastroesophageal reflux in steroid-dependent asthmatic youths. Pediatrics. 1979;63(2):207–12.

85. Euler AR, Byrne WJ, Ament ME, Fonkalsrud EW, Strobel CT, Siegel SC, et al. Recurrent pulmonary disease in children: a complication of gastroesophageal reflux. Pediatrics. 1979;63(1):47–51.

86. Martin ME, Grunstein MM, Larsen GL. The relationship of gastroesophageal reflux to nocturnal wheezing in children with asthma. Ann Allergy. 1982;49(6):318–22.

87. Buts JP, Barudi C, Moulin D, Claus D, Cornu G, Otte JB. Prevalence and treatment of silent gastro-oesophageal reflux in children with recurrent respiratory disorders. Eur J Pediatr. 1986;145(5):396–400.

88. Gustafsson PM, Kjellman NI, Tibbling L. Bronchial asthma and acid reflux into the distal and proximal oesophagus. Arch Dis Child. 1990;65(11):1255–8.

89. Andze GO, Brandt ML, St Vil D, Bensoussan AL, Blanchard H. Diagnosis and treatment of gastroesophageal reflux in 500 children with respiratory symptoms: the value of pH monitoring. J Pediatr Surg. 1991;26(3):295–9.

90. Boulet LP, Boulay MÈ. Asthma-related comorbidities. Expert Rev Respir Med. 2011;5(3):377–93.

91. Gibson PG, Henry RL, Coughlan JL. Gastro-oesophageal reflux treatment for asthma in adults and children. Cochrane Database Syst Rev. 2003;2:CD001496.

92. Mastronarde JG, Anthonisen NR, Castro M, Holbrook JT, Leone FT, Teague WG, et al. Efficacy of esomeprazole for treatment of poorly controlled asthma. N Engl J Med. 2009;360(15):1487–99.

93. Kiljander TO, Harding SM, Field SK, Stein MR, Nelson HS, Ekelund J, et al. Effects of esomeprazole 40 mg twice daily on asthma: a randomized placebo-controlled trial. Am J Respir Crit Care Med. 2006;173(10):1091–7.

94. Littner MR, Leung FW, Ballard ED, Huang B, Samra NK. Effects of 24 weeks of lansoprazole therapy on asthma symptoms, exacerbations, quality of life, and pulmonary function in adult asthmatic patients with acid reflux symptoms. Chest. 2005;128(3):1128–35.

95. Kiljander TO, Junghard O, Beckman O, Lind T. Effect of esomeprazole 40 mg once or twice daily on asthma: a randomized, placebo-controlled study. Am J Respir Crit Care Med. 2010;181(10):1042–8.

96. Sontag SJ, O'Connell S, Khandelwal S, Greenlee H, Schnell T, Nemchausky B, et al. Asthmatics with gastroesophageal reflux: long term results of a randomized trial of medical and surgical antireflux therapies. Am J Gastroenterol. 2003;98(5):987–99.

97. Herzig SJ, Howell MD, Ngo LH, Marcantonio ER. Acid-suppressive medication use and the risk for hospital-acquired pneumonia. JAMA. 2009;301(20):2120–8.

98. Mcdonald EG, Milligan J, Frenette C, Lee TC. Continuous proton pump inhibitor therapy and the associated risk of recurrent Clostridium difficile infection. JAMA Intern Med. 2015;175(5):784–91.

99. Yu EW, Bauer SR, Bain PA, Bauer DC. Proton pump inhibitors and risk of fractures: a meta-

analysis of 11 international studies. Am J Med. 2011;124(6):519–26.

100. Taveras EM, Rifas-Shiman SL, Camargo CA Jr, Gold DR, Litonjua AA, Oken E, et al. Higher adiposity in infancy associated with recurrent wheeze in a prospective cohort of children. J Allergy Clin Immunol. 2008;121(5):1161–1166.e3.

101. Flaherman V, Rutherford GW. A meta-analysis of the effect of high weight on asthma. Arch Dis Child. 2006;91(4):334–9.

102. Guh DP, Zhang W, Bansback N, Amarsi Z, Birmingham CL, Anis AH. The incidence of co-morbidities related to obesity and overweight: a systematic review and meta-analysis. BMC Public Health. 2009;9:88.

103. Visness CM, London SJ, Daniels JL, Kaufman JS, Yeatts KB, Siega-Riz AM, et al. Association of childhood obesity with atopic and nonatopic asthma: results from the National Health and Nutrition Examination Survey 1999-2006. J Asthma. 2010;47(7):822–9.

104. Shore SA. Obesity and asthma: implications for treatment. Curr Opin Pulm Med. 2007;13(1):56–62.

105. Aaron SD, Fergusson D, Dent R, Chen Y, Vandemheen KL, Dales RE. Effect of weight reduction on respiratory function and airway reactivity in obese women. Chest. 2004;125(6):2046–52.

106. Maniscalco M, Zedda A, Faraone S, Cerbone MR, Cristiano S, Giardiello C, et al. Weight loss and asthma control in severely obese asthmatic females. Respir Med. 2008;102(1):102–8.

107. Eneli IU, Skybo T, Camargo CA. Weight loss and asthma: a systematic review. Thorax. 2008;63(8):671–6.

108. Shore SA. Obesity and asthma: possible mechanisms. J Allergy Clin Immunol. 2008;121(5):1087–93.

109. Lessard A, Turcotte H, Cormier Y, Boulet LP. Obesity and asthma: a specific phenotype? Chest. 2008;134(2):317–23.

110. Saint-pierre P, Bourdin A, Chanez P, Daures JP, Godard P. Are overweight asthmatics more difficult to control? Allergy. 2006;61(1):79–84.

111. Boulet LP, Franssen E. Influence of obesity on response to fluticasone with or without sal-meterol in moderate asthma. Respir Med. 2007;101(11):2240–7.

112. Pakhale S, Doucette S, Vandemheen K, Boulet LP, McIvor RA, Fitzgerald JM, et al. A comparison of obese and nonobese people with asthma: exploring an asthma-obesity interaction. Chest. 2010;137(6):1316–23.

113. Yigla M, Tov N, Solomonov A, Rubin AH, Harlev D. Difficult-to-control asthma and obstructive sleep apnea. J Asthma. 2003;40(8):865–71.

114. Young T, Palta M, Dempsey J, Skatrud J, Weber S, Badr S. The occurrence of sleep-disordered breathing among middle-aged adults. N Engl J Med. 1993;328(17):1230–5.

115. Mehra R, Redline S. Sleep apnea: a proinflammatory disorder that coaggregates with obesity. J Allergy Clin Immunol. 2008;121(5):1096–102.

116. Chan CS, Woolcock AJ, Sullivan CE. Nocturnal asthma: role of snoring and obstructive sleep apnea. Am Rev Respir Dis. 1988;137(6):1502–4.

117. Ciftci TU, Ciftci B, Guven SF, Kokturk O, Turktas H. Effect of nasal continuous positive airway pressure in uncontrolled nocturnal asthmatic patients with obstructive sleep apnea syndrome. Respir Med. 2005;99(5):529–34.

118. Lafond C, Sériès F, Lemière C. Impact of CPAP on asthmatic patients with obstructive sleep apnoea. Eur Respir J. 2007;29(2):307–11.

119. ten Brinke A, Ouwerkerk ME, Bel EH, Spinhoven P. Similar psychological characteristics in mild and severe asthma. J Psychosom Res. 2001;50(1):7–10.

120. Kuehn BM. Asthma linked to psychiatric disorders. JAMA. 2008;299(2):158–60.

121. Nouwen A, Freeston MH, Labbé R, Boulet LP. Psychological factors associated with emergency room visits among asthmatic patients. Behav Modif. 1999;23(2):217–33.

122. Lehrer P, Feldman J, Giardino N, Song HS, Schmaling K. Psychological aspects of asthma. J Consult Clin Psychol. 2002;70(3):691–711.

123. Feldman JM, Siddique MI, Morales E, Kaminski B, Lu SE, Lehrer PM. Psychiatric disorders and asthma outcomes among high-risk inner-city patients. Psychosom Med. 2005;67(6):989–96.

124. Lavoie KL, Bacon SL, Barone S, Cartier A, Ditto B, Labrecque M. What is worse for asthma control and quality of life: depressive disorders, anxiety disorders, or both? Chest. 2006;130(4):1039–47.

125. Heaney LG, Conway E, Kelly C, Gamble J. Prevalence of psychiatric morbidity in a difficult asthma population: relationship to asthma outcome. Respir Med. 2005;99(9):1152–9.

126. Nowobilski R, Furgał M, Czyz P, De Barbaro B, Polczyk R, Bochenek G, et al. Psychopathology and personality factors modify the perception of dyspnea in asthmatics. J Asthma. 2007;44(3):203–7.

127. Katon W, Lozano P, Russo J, Mccauley E, Richardson L, Bush T. The prevalence of DSM-IV anxiety and depressive disorders in youth with asthma compared with controls. J Adolesc Health. 2007;41(5):455–63.

128. Wainwright NW, Surtees PG, Wareham NJ, Harrison BD. Psychosocial factors and incident asthma hospital admissions in the EPIC-Norfolk cohort study. Allergy. 2007;62(5):554–60.

129. Forbes L, Harvey S, Newson R, Jarvis D, Luczynska C, Price J, et al. Risk factors for accident and emergency (A&E) attendance for asthma in inner city children. Thorax. 2007;62(10):855–60.

130. Dahlem NW, Kinsman RA, Horton DJ. Panic-fear in asthma: requests for as-needed medications in relation to pulmonary function measurements. J Allergy Clin Immunol. 1977;60(5):295–300.

131. Rimington LD, Davies DH, Lowe D, Pearson MG. Relationship between anxiety, depression, and morbidity in adult asthma patients. Thorax. 2001;56(4):266–71.

132. Yorke J, Fleming SL, Shuldham C. A systematic review of psychological interventions for children with asthma. Pediatr Pulmonol. 2007;42(2):114–24.

133. Lehrer PM, Karavidas MK, Lu SE, Feldman J, Kranitz L, Abraham S, et al. Psychological treatment of comorbid asthma and panic disorder: a pilot study. J Anxiety Disord. 2008;22(4):671–83.

134. Yorke J, Fleming SL, Shuldham C. Psychological interventions for adults with asthma: a systematic review. Respir Med. 2007;101(1):1–14.

135. Husein OF, Husein TN, Gardner R, Chiang T, Larson DG, Obert K, et al. Formal psychological testing in patients with paradoxical vocal fold dysfunction. Laryngoscope. 2008;118(4):740–7.

136. Thomas M, Mckinley RK, Freeman E, Foy C, Price D. The prevalence of dysfunctional breathing in adults in the community with and without asthma. Prim Care Respir J. 2005;14(2):78–82.

137. Thomas M, Mckinley RK, Freeman E, Foy C, Prodger P, Price D. Breathing retraining for dysfunctional breathing in asthma: a randomised controlled trial. Thorax. 2003;58(2):110–5.

138. Newman KB, Mason UG, Schmaling KB. Clinical features of vocal cord dysfunction. Am J Respir Crit Care Med. 1995;152(4 Pt 1):1382–6.

139. Ibrahim WH, Gheriani HA, Almohamed AA, Raza T. Paradoxical vocal cord motion disorder: past, present and future. Postgrad Med J. 2007;83(977):164–72.

140. Balkissoon R, Kenn K. Asthma: vocal cord dysfunction (VCD) and other dysfunctional breathing disorders. Semin Respir Crit Care Med. 2012;33(6):595–605.

141. Traister RS, Fajt ML, Landsittel D, Petrov AA. A novel scoring system to distinguish vocal cord dysfunction from asthma. J Allergy Clin Immunol Pract. 2014;2(1):65–9.

142. Greenberger PA. Allergic bronchopulmonary aspergillosis. Allergy Asthma Proc. 2012;33:S61–3.

143. Denning DW, Pleuvry A, Cole DC. Global burden of allergic bronchopulmonary aspergillosis with asthma and its complication chronic pulmonary aspergillosis in adults. Med Mycol. 2013;51(4):361–70.

144. Schwartz HJ, Greenberger PA. The prevalence of allergic bronchopulmonary aspergillosis in patients with asthma, determined by serologic and radiologic criteria in patients at risk. J Lab Clin Med. 1991;117:138–42.

145. Basich JE, Graves TS, Baz MN, Scanlon G, Hoffmann RG, Patterson R, et al. Allergic bronchopulmonary aspergillosis in corticosteroid-dependent asthmatics. J Allergy Clin Immunol. 1981;68:98–102.

146. Becker JW, Burke W, McDonald G, Greenberger PA, Henderson WR, Aitken ML, et al. Prevalence of allergic bronchopulmonary aspergillosis and atopy in adult patients with cystic fibrosis. Chest. 1996;109:1536–40.

147. Hinson KFW, Moon AJ, Plummer NS. Bronchopulmonary aspergillosis. A review and a report of eight new cases. Thorax. 1952;7:317–33.

148. Patterson R, Golbert TM. Hypersensitivity disease of the lung. Univ Mich Med Cent J. 1968;34:8–11.

149. Greenberger PA, Patterson R. Allergic bronchopulmonary aspergillosis: model of bronchopulmonary disease with defined serologic, radiologic, pathologic and clinical findings from asthma to fatal destructive lung disease. Chest. 1987;91:165S–71S.

150. Maurya V, Gugnani HC, Sarma PU, Madan T, Shah A. Sensitization to Aspergillus antigens and occurrence of allergic bronchopulmonary aspergillosis in patients with asthma. Chest. 2005;127:1252–9.

151. Zureik M, Neukirch C, Leynaert B, Liard R, Bousquet J, Neukirch F, et al. Sensitisation to airborne moulds and severity of asthma: cross sectional study from European Community respiratory health survey. BMJ. 2002;325(7361):411–4.

152. Virnig C, Bush RK. Allergic bronchopulmonary aspergillosis: a US perspective. Curr Opin Pulm Med. 2007;13:67–71.

153. Geller DE, Kaplowitz H, Light MJ, Colin AA. Allergic bronchopulmonary aspergillosis in cystic fibrosis: reported prevalence, regional distribution, and patient characteristics. Chest. 1999;116:639–46.

154. Greenberger PA, Bush RK, Demain JG, Luong A, Slavin RG, Knutsen AP, et al. Allergic bronchopulmonary aspergillosis. J Allergy Clin Immunol Pract. 2014;2:703–8.

155. Gibson GP. Allergic bronchopulmonary aspergillosis. Semin Respir Crit Care Med. 2006;27:185–91.

156. Wark PA, Gibson PG. Allergic bronchopulmonary aspergillosis: new concepts of pathogenesis and treatment. Respirology. 2001;6:1–7.

157. Lazarus AA, Thilagar B, McKay SA. Allergic bronchopulmonary aspergillosis. Dis Mon. 2008;54:547–64.

158. Moss RB. Pathophysiology and immunology of allergic bronchopulmonary aspergillosis. Med Mycol. 2005;43(suppl1):S203–6.

159. Patterson K, Strek ME. Allergic bronchopulmonary aspergillosis. Proc Am Thorac Soc. 2010;7:237–44.

160. Rosenberg M, Patterson R, Mintzer R, Cooper BJ, Roberts M, Harris KE. Clinical and immunologic criteria for the diagnosis of allergic bronchopulmonary aspergillosis. Ann Intern Med. 1977;86:405–14.

161. Patterson R, Greenberger PA, Halwig JM. Allergic bronchopulmonary aspergillosis: natural history and classification of early disease by serologic and roentgenographic studies. Arch Intern Med. 1986;146:916–8.

162. Jacoby B, Longbottom JL, Pepys J. The uptake of Aspergillus fumigatus protein by serum IgG antibody from patients with pulmonary aspergillosis. Clin Allergy. 1977;7:117–25.

163. O'Driscoll BR, Powell G, Chew F, Niven RM, Miles JF, Vyas A, et al. Comparison of skin prick tests with specific serum immunoglobulin E in the diagnosis of fungal sensitization in patients with severe asthma. Clin Exp Allergy. 2009;39:1677–83.

164. Fairs A, Agbetile J, Hargadon B, Bourne M, Monteiro WR, Brightling CE, et al. IgE sensitization to Aspergillus fumigatus is associated with reduced lung function in asthma. Am J Respir Crit Care Med. 2010;182:1362–8.

165. Agarwal R. Allergic bronchopulmonary aspergillosis. Chest. 2009;135:805–26.

166. Greenberger PA, Miller TP, Roberts M, Smith LL. Allergic bronchopulmonary aspergillosis in patients with and without bronchiectasis. Ann Allergy. 1993;70:333–8.

167. Greenberger PA. Allergic bronchopulmonary aspergillosis. J Allergy Clin Immunol. 2002;110(5):685–92.

168. Slavin RG, Hutcheson PS, Chauhan B, Bellone CJ. An overview of allergic bronchopulmonary aspergillosis with some new insights. Allergy Asthma Proc. 2004;25(6):395–9.

169. Casaulta C, Fluckiger S, Crameri R, Blaser K, Schoeni MH. Time course of antibody response to recombinant Aspergillus fumigatus antigens in cystic fibrosis with and without ABPA. Pediatr Allergy Immunol. 2005;16:217–25.

170. Agarwal R, Aggarwal AN, Gupta D, Jindal SK. Aspergillus hypersensitivity and allergic bronchopulmonary aspergillosis in patients with bronchial asthma: systematic review and meta-analysis. Int J Tuberc Lung Dis. 2009;13(8):936–44.

171. Agarwal R, Gupta D, Aggarwal AN, Saxena AK, Saikia B, Chakrabarti A, et al. Clinical significance of decline in serum IgE levels in allergic bronchopulmonary aspergillosis. Respir Med. 2010;104:204–10.

172. Panchal N, Bhagat R, Pant C, Shah A. Allergic bronchopulmonary aspergillosis: the spectrum of computed tomography appearances. Respir Med. 1997;91:213–9.

173. Menzies D, Holmes L, McCumesky G, Prys-Picard C, Niven R. Aspergillus sensitization is associated with airflow limitation and bronchiectasis in severe asthma. Allergy. 2011;66:679–85.

174. Agarwal R, Gupta D, Aggarwal AN, Behera D, Jindal SK. Allergic bronchopulmonary aspergillosis: lessons from 126 patients attending a chest clinic in north India. Chest. 2006;130:442–8.

175. Vlahakis NE, Aksamit TR. Diagnosis and treatment of allergic bronchopulmonary aspergillosis. Mayo Clin Proc. 2001;76:930–8.

176. Stevens DA, Schwartz HJ, Lee JY, Moskovitz BL, Jerome DC, Catanzaro A, et al. A randomized trial of itraconazole in allergic bronchopulmonary aspergillosis. N Engl J Med. 2000;342:756–62.

177. Wark PA, Hensley MJ, Saltos N, Boyle MJ, Toneguzzi RC, Epid GD, et al. Anti-inflammatory effect of itraconazole in stable allergic bronchopulmonary aspergillosis: a randomized controlled trial. J Allergy Clin Immunol. 2003;111:952–7.

178. Wark PA, Gibson PG, Wilson AJ. Azoles for allergic bronchopulmonary aspergillosis associated with asthma. Cochrane Database Syst Rev. 2004;3:CD001108.

179. Glackin L, Leen G, Elnazir B, Greally P. Voriconazole in the treatment of allergic bronchopulmonary aspergillosis in cystic fibro-sis. Irish Med J. 2009;102:29.

180. Tillie-Leblond I, Germaud P, Leroyer C, Tétu L, Girard F, Devouassoux G, et al. Allergic bronchopulmonary aspergillosis and omalizumab. Allergy. 2011;66(9):1254–6.

181. Gilbert G. Unusual idiosyncrasy to aspirin. JAMA. 1911;56:1262.

182. Widal MF, Abrami P, Lenmoyez J. Anaphylaxie et idiosyncrasie. Presse Med. 1922;30:189–93.

183. Samter M, Beers RF. Intolerance to aspirin. Clinical studies and consideration of its pathogenesis. Ann Intern Med. 1968;68(5):975–83.

184. Berges-gimeno MP, Simon RA, Stevenson DD. The natural history and clinical characteristics of aspirin-exacerbated respiratory disease. Ann Allergy Asthma Immunol. 2002;89(5):474–8.

185. Pfaar O, Klimek L. Aspirin desensitization in aspirin intolerance: update on current standards and recent improvements. Curr Opin Allergy Clin Immunol. 2006;6(3):161–6.

186. Rajan JP, Wineinger NE, Stevenson DD, White AA. Prevalence of aspirin-exacerbated respiratory disease among asthmatic patients: a meta-analysis of the literature. J Allergy Clin Immunol. 2015;135(3):676–81.e1.

187. Szczeklik A, Nizankowska E, Duplaga M. Natural history of aspirin-induced asthma. AIANE Investigators. European Network on Aspirin-Induced Asthma. Eur Respir J. 2000;16(3):432–6.

188. Stevenson DD, Szczeklik A. Clinical and pathologic perspectives on aspirin sensitivity and asthma. J Allergy Clin Immunol. 2006;118(4):773–86.

189. Miller B, Mirakian R, Gane S, Larco J, Sannah AA, Darby Y, et al. Nasal lysine aspirin challenge in the diagnosis of aspirin—exacerbated respiratory disease: asthma and rhinitis. Clin Exp Allergy. 2013;43(8):874–80.

190. Gamboa P, Sanz ML, Caballero MR, Urrutia I, Antépara I, Esparza R, et al. The flow-cytometric determination of basophil activation induced by aspirin and other non-steroidal anti-inflammatory drugs (NSAIDs) is useful for in vitro diagnosis of the NSAID hypersensitivity syndrome. Clin Exp Allergy. 2004;34(9):1448–57.

191. White A, Bigby T, Stevenson D. Intranasal ketorolac challenge for the diagnosis of aspirin-exacerbated respiratory disease. Ann Allergy Asthma Immunol. 2006;97(2):190–5.

192. Szczeklik A, Sanak M, Nizankowska-mogilnicka E, Kiełbasa B. Aspirin intolerance and the cyclooxygenase-leukotriene pathways. Curr Opin Pulm Med. 2004;10(1):51–6.

193. Sousa AR, Parikh A, Scadding G, Corrigan CJ, Lee TH. Leukotriene-receptor expression on nasal mucosal inflammatory cells in aspirin-sensitive rhinosinusitis. N Engl J Med. 2002;347(19):1493–9.

194. Sestini P, Armetti L, Gambaro G, Pieroni MG, Refini RM, Sala A, et al. Inhaled PGE2 prevents aspirin-induced bronchoconstriction and urinary LTE4 excretion in aspirin-sensitive asthma. Am J Respir Crit Care Med. 1996;153(2):572–5.

195. Schäfer D, Schmid M, Göde UC, Baenkler HW. Dynamics of eicosanoids in peripheral blood cells during bronchial provocation in aspirin-intolerant asthmatics. Eur Respir J. 1999;13(3):638–46.

196. Cowburn AS, Sladek K, Soja J, Adamek L, Nizankowska E, Szczeklik A, et al. Overexpression of leukotriene C4 synthase in bronchial biopsies from patients with aspirin-intolerant asthma. J Clin Invest. 1998;101(4):834–46.

197. Higashi N, Taniguchi M, Mita H, Kawagishi Y, Ishii T, Higashi A, et al. Clinical features of asthmatic patients with increased urinary leukotriene E4 excretion (hyperleukotrienuria): involvement of chronic hyperplastic rhinosinusitis with nasal polyposis. J Allergy Clin Immunol. 2004;113(2):277–83.

198. Macy E, Bernstein JA, Castells MC, Gawchik SM, Lee TH, Settipane RA, et al. Aspirin challenge and desensitization for aspirin-exacerbated respiratory disease: a practice paper. Ann Allergy Asthma Immunol. 2007;98(2):172–4.

199. Simon RA. Treatment of patients with respiratory reactions to aspirin and nonsteroidal anti-inflammatory drugs. Curr Allergy Asthma Rep. 2004;4(2):139–43.

200. Szczeklik A, Nizankowska E, Bochenek G, Nagraba K, Mejza F, Swierczynska M. Safety of a specific COX-2 inhibitor in aspirin-induced asthma. Clin Exp Allergy. 2001;31(2):219–25.

201. Morales DR, Lipworth BJ, Guthrie B, Jackson C, Donnan PT, Santiago VH. Safety risks for patients with aspirin-exacerbated respiratory disease after acute exposure to selective nonsteroidal anti-inflammatory drugs and COX-2 inhibitors: meta-analysis of controlled clinical trials. J Allergy Clin Immunol. 2014;134(1):40–5.

202. Settipane RA, Schrank PJ, Simon RA, Mathison DA, Christiansen SC, Stevenson DD. Prevalence of cross-sensitivity with acetaminophen in aspirin-sensitive asthmatic subjects. J Allergy Clin Immunol. 1995;96(4):480–5.

203. Dahlén B, Nizankowska E, Szczeklik A, Zetterström O, Bochenek G, Kumlin M, et al. Benefits from adding the 5-lipoxygenase inhibitor zileuton to conventional therapy in aspirin-intolerant asthmatics. Am J Respir Crit Care Med. 1998;157:1187–94.

204. Dahlén SE, Malmström K, Nizankowska E, Dahlén B, Kuna P, Kowalski M, et al. Improvement of aspirin-intolerant asthma by montelukast, a leukotriene antagonist. Am J Respir Crit Care Med. 2002;165:9–14.

205. Berges-Gimeno MP, Simon RA, Stevenson DD. Long-term treatment with aspirin desensitization in asthmatic patients with aspirin-exacerbated respiratory disease. J Allergy Clin Immunol. 2003;111:180–6.

206. Lee RU, White AA, Ding D, Dursun AB, Woessner KM, Simon RA, et al. Use of intranasal ketorolac and modified oral aspirin challenge for desensitization of aspirin-exacerbated respiratory disease. Ann Allergy Asthma Immunol. 2010;105(2):130–5.

207. Nakamura H, Kawasaki M, Higuchi Y, Takahashi S. Effects of sinus surgery on asthma in aspirin triad patients. Acta Otolaryngol. 1999;119(5):592–8.

208. Loehrl TA, Ferre RM, Toohill RJ, Smith TL. Long-term asthma outcomes after endoscopic sinus surgery in aspirin triad patients. Am J Otolaryngol. 2006;27(3):154–60.

Part II

Pathobiology of Severe Asthma

Pathogenesis of Severe Asthma

3

So Ri Kim

3.1 Structural Abnormalities and Airway Remodeling

Airway remodeling encompasses various structural alterations of airways in asthmatic patients and involves a wide array of pathophysiologic features, including epithelial changes, increased smooth muscle mass, increased numbers of activated fibroblasts/myofibroblasts, subepithelial fibrosis, and vascular changes. In addition, airway remodeling is a representative pathologic hallmark of asthmatic severity, and these structural changes are speculated to be one of the factors that make it difficult to treat asthmatic patients and therefore may be a target for future therapies of severe asthma [1, 2].

3.1.1 Alterations of Bronchial Epithelium

Bronchial epithelium is composed of two major airway epithelial cell types, ciliated and secretory cells and is critical for preserving airway patency and defending against inhaled pathogens and allergens. Epithelial alterations in asthmatic

patients include shedding of the epithelium, loss of ciliated cells, goblet cell hyperplasia, and upregulation of growth factors, cytokines, and chemokines. In particular, the epithelium in severe asthma is reported to be thicker than in mild-to-moderate asthma [3], with altered proliferation, apoptosis, and release of pro-inflammatory factors [4]. These epithelial alterations appear to be caused by two ways: (1) ongoing epithelial injury due to infectious agents, allergens, or inhaled particulates and (2) persistent host immune responses (i.e., damage-associated molecular patterns [DAMPs] or danger signals). Direct structural interruption of bronchial epithelium including loss of epithelial integrity, disruption of tight junctions, impairment of barrier function, and cell death induces impaired epithelial permeability playing as a prerequisite for antigen caption and presentation by the surrounding dendritic cells (DCs) [5]. In addition, these epithelial injury and dysfunction may correlate with asthma severity [6–9]. Recent studies have demonstrated that mechanical stress such as bronchoconstriction, a crucial characteristic of asthma, initiates the activation of signaling cascades and the release of fibrotic and inflammatory mediators in airway epithelial cells [10–12]. Moreover, the compressive effect of bronchospasm also causes mature airway epithelial cells to move in collective fluid-like swirls (unjamming), whereas otherwise they are solid-like and virtually immobile (jamming). In bronchial epithelium from asthmatics, the recovery

S.R. Kim
Division of Respiratory Medicine and Allergy,
Department of Internal Medicine,
Chonbuk National University Medical School,
Jeonju 54907, South Korea
e-mail: sori@jbnu.ac.kr

© Springer Nature Singapore Pte Ltd. 2018
Y.C. Lee et al. (eds.), *Severe Asthma*, https://doi.org/10.1007/978-981-10-1998-2_3

into jamming phase is delayed compare to normal subjects [13]. These cellular motilities appear also to contribute to the defective asthmatic epithelial function and integrity. As for ciliated epithelial cells, although relatively few studies have been performed than secretory cells, decreased ciliary beat frequency and increases in abnormal ciliary beating patterns and ciliary ultrastructural defects have been reported in individuals with asthma compared with healthy controls [14]. In addition, these abnormalities were more pronounced in severe asthma. Ciliary abnormalities were accompanied by increases in the numbers of dead cells and evidence of loss of epithelial structural integrity, which suggests that ciliary dysfunction may be a consequence of a generalized epithelial injury and can be one of contributing factors to develop severe asthma.

Asthmatic airway epithelial cells respond to various host and environmental stimuli through participating in diverse immune and inflammatory processes. First, asthmatic airway epithelium secretes the cytokines TSLP, IL-25, and IL-33, which act on subepithelial DCs, mast cells, and innate lymphoid cells (ILCs) to recruit both innate and adaptive hematopoietic cells and initiate the release of Th2 cytokines [15–19]. In addition, a recent human study has reported that in patients with severe asthma and persistent eosinophilia, the number of ILC2s in blood and airways is substantially increased compared with mild asthma suggesting that the role of epithelial-derived cytokines such as TSLP, IL-25, and IL-33 in recruiting ILC2 is a more crucial component of the pathogenesis of eosinophilic severe asthma rather than mild asthma [20]. On the other hand, under stressful conditions including cigarette smoking and lipopolysaccharide (LPS) stimulation, bronchial epithelium seems to induce neutrophilic airway inflammation, which is another phenotype of severe asthma through increased secretions of chemoattractants for neutrophils including IL-17A, IL-6, IL-8, and CXCL8 [21–23]. And the extent of the production of these mediators is correlated positively with asthma severity [4]. Moreover, in patients with chronic rhinosinusitis and nasal polyp as well as those with severe asthma, neutrophils act as a major source of oncostatin M, an epithelial barrier disrupting cytokine participating in the pathogenesis of severe asthma [24]. Meanwhile, lipoxins (LXs) are a natural anti-inflammatory factor produced at the inflamed tissue site to downregulate inflammation and to promote its resolution [25]. Levels of LXA4 were reduced in samples from patients with severe asthma compared with levels seen in patients with mild asthma [25, 26]. These findings suggest that bronchial epithelial cells are associated with various phenotypes of severe asthmatic inflammation as an immune and inflammatory modulator.

Although abnormalities in mucus are not limited to severe asthma and exacerbations because an increase in mucous metaplasia is seen even in individuals with stable, mild-to-moderate asthma [27], more increased amount of mucin production in epithelium and tenacious and viscous property of mucus are implicated in the development of severe asthma [4, 28]. A variety of stimuli and signaling pathways have been shown to regulate mucin production and secretion in airway epithelial cells. Known MUC5AC inducers are usually signaled through STAT6/SAM domain-containing prostate-derived Ets factor (SPDEF) activation, phosphoinositide 3-kinase (PI3K)-nuclear factor of activated T cells (NFAT) pathway, and FoxA2 inhibition under IL-13 receptor activation or by ErbB receptor agonists (i.e., EGF, TGF-α, amphiregulin) through HIF-1 and MAPK pathways [23, 29, 30]. In addition, glucocorticoids are not sufficient to suppress IL-13-induced goblet cell hyperplasia [31]. Based on these contentions, many signaling pathways have evaluated the potential of drug target to resolve the pathologic mucus production in steroid-resistant severe asthma.

3.1.2 Proliferation and Hypertrophy of Airway Smooth Muscle (ASM)

Airway remodeling is considered to be the cardinal feature leading onto the development and persistence of airflow obstruction. In particular, the increase in ASM content is believed to explain the majority of airway luminal narrowing and the permanent reduction of the airway caliber in severe asthma; whether this increase in ASM mass is due to hyperplasia, hypertrophy, or both remains uncertain [32, 33]. In fact, ASM mass is increased in severe asthma compared to mild-to-moderate asthma or chronic bronchitis [32, 34–37], suggesting that ASM increased is related to asthma severity. In view of the biology of ASM, the contractile property also contributes to induce airway obstruction in asthmatics and other airway disorders compared to normal subjects, however, the differences of contractile strength or its related protein expression between mild-to-moderate asthma and severe asthma are somewhat controversial. Quantitative analytic data using human bronchial biopsy samples from mild, moderate, and severe persistent asthmatics showed that the intensity of MLCK expression was further amplified in patients with severe persistent asthma, while the protein expressions of α-actin and the smooth muscle myosin heavy-chain isoforms were similar in patients with asthma from all groups [32]. Given that many immune and inflammatory mediators such as TNF-α, IL-17, and IL-13 have been shown to increase ASM contractility and at the same time these mediators are closely associated with asthma severity and the pathogenesis of severe asthma [38–40], ASM contractility is expected to contribute to the pathogenesis of severe asthma, and this field still remains as unanswered completely with needs more well-designed future studies.

Several mechanisms may explain an increased ASM mass in asthma. First, the presence of extracellular matrix (ECM) deposition such as collagen in and around ASM bundles may contribute to the overall increase in the ASM content [41, 42]. However, Benayoun et al. have reported that the increased ASM cell size observed in patients with severe persistent asthma reflects true cell hypertrophy and not merely the presence of collagen deposit within ASM cells [32]. The other mechanism is the participation of fibromyocytes in forming ASM bundles [43]. This concept is also ambiguous in reflecting

asthma severity since a quantitative analytic data revealed that α-actin-positive cells (i.e., myofibroblast or fibromyoblast) did not vary significantly between the three asthma groups of intermittent, mild-to-moderate persistent, and severe persistent asthma [32]. Although relatively little information has released on the role and the related mechanisms of ASM remodeling in the severe asthma, a recent study enrolled the patients with mild-to-moderate asthma and severe asthma has demonstrated that symptoms in patients with severe asthma with increased ASM area are less controlled by maximal therapy than those with lower ASM area. Interestingly, ASM enlargement was associated with increased expression of PAR-2 and high BAL levels of their ligands, particularly mast cell tryptase and KLK14 [44]. These findings suggest that increased ASM mass characterizes the patients with severe asthma with poor symptom control and the delicate mechanisms for the increased ASM mass in severe asthma must be defined for the control of severe asthma.

3.1.3 Fibrosis, Subepithelial Thickening, and Alternation of ECM

Subepithelial thickening of airways has been observed in asthma of all severities, with deposition of collagens, fibronectin, tenascin, and proteoglycans [45–48]. The results are not always consistent, but the majority of studies showed that severe asthmatics have thicker subepithelial layers compared to those with mild disease [3, 34, 35, 49–54]. In fact, fibrocytes are increased in blood and in smooth muscle bundles in asthmatics with fixed airway obstruction and/or severe asthma [55, 56]. There is still debate on whether the subepithelial thickening is gradually developed with time as a consequence of repeated episodes of allergen exposure and bouts of acute inflammation or the thickening is already formed at early stage of the natural course of severe asthma. Many previous studies have demonstrated that chronic airway inflammation has been considered to be the primary abnormality in asthma and remodeling a secondary consequence [57, 58]. On the other hand, Payne et al. and others have reported that subepithelial thickening of the bronchial reticular layer is an early feature of severe asthma in children and appears to be a characteristic of the eosinophilic phenotype [54, 59]. In addition, patients with severe asthmatics also have increased expression of TGF-β isoforms and collagen deposition as compared to mild asthmatics, again in association with eosinophilic asthma, with evidence for remodeling in the peripheral airways as well [60, 61]. Moreover, increased production and altered composition of extracellular matrix in the small airways are characteristics of fatal asthma [61]. To sum up, these reports suggest that subepithelial thickening, ECM alterations, and subepithelial fibrosis are important features of severe asthma. Supporting these observations, recent studies have revealed the related mechanisms; IL-33 promotes airway remodeling in patients with steroid-resistant asthma, specifically through increasing collagen secretions from airway fibroblasts [62]. Furthermore, in severe asthma with fungal sensitization (SAFS), IL-33 and MMP-9 are more increased in airways than the levels in non-SAFS [63]. Taken together, alterations of subepithelial layer of airways are one of pathogenic characteristics of severe asthma in which there may be a distinct inducer from non-severe asthma.

3.1.4 Vascularity and Vascular Permeability

A number of studies have shown a relationship between the increased bronchial vascular remodeling and the severity of asthmatic disease [64–68]. Bronchial vascular remodeling in asthma includes vasodilation, increased blood flow, angiogenesis, and increased vascular permeability. In addition, most inflammatory mediators cause bronchial vasodilation [69–71]. It is also postulated that the increase in bronchial microcirculation and airway blood flow amplifies inflammatory responses by acting as a gateway to the subepithelium for inflammatory cells,

although some reports have demonstrated that increased airway blood flow may play a role in removing inflammatory mediators from airways [72]. Moreover, the increase in the number and size of vessels can contribute to the thickening of the airway wall, which in turn may lead to critical narrowing of the bronchial lumen, as bronchial smooth muscle contraction occurs [73]. Among various angiogenic growth factors, vascular endothelial growth factor (VEGF) and angiopoietin-1 (Ang-1) have been reported to play the most relevant roles in vascular changes in the airways of asthmatic subjects [74–76]. Indeed, in asthmatic patients, the overproduction of VEGF is implicated in asthma exacerbation, and the circulating VEGF levels were significantly inversely correlated with the percent predicted FEV1 suggesting that measurement of either plasma or serum VEGF level can be a valid index of asthma severity [77, 78]. In addition, Lee et al. have demonstrated that mast cells which amplify the inflammation and contribute to development of airway remodeling modulate vascular permeability through the regulation of PI3K–HIF-1α–VEGF axis in allergic asthma [79]. Sequentially, inhibition of VEGF and/or PI3K/Akt pathway attenuates peribronchial fibrosis and subepithelial collagen deposition by reduction of transforming growth factor (TGF)-β1 expression in bronchial epithelial cells of asthmatic mice [80]. In mice with chronic inhaled ovalbumin (OVA) exposure, potent antioxidants attenuate OVA-induced airway remodeling including subepithelial fibrosis through inhibition of TGF-β1 production and PI3K/VEGF pathway [81]. Among class I PI3K isoforms, PI3K-δ isoform is known to contribute to the development of steroid-resistant asthma [82]. More interestingly, selective PI3K-δ inhibition reduces vascular permeability and expression of VEGF through regulation of HIF-1α and HIF-2α levels of the lung, specifically in bronchial epithelium [83, 84]. Taken together, these contentions suggest that vascular abnormalities in asthmatic airways are more prominent in severe asthma and VEGF-PI3K-δ relationship is a valuable target for the novel therapeutic agents through the modulation of vascular remodeling.

3.2 Corticosteroid Resistance and Its Molecular Mechanisms

The definition of severe asthma has primarily been based upon corticosteroid responsiveness and clinical symptoms. Thus, to date, several molecular mechanisms of corticosteroid resistance have been elucidated in severe asthmatic patients providing the therapeutic potential targets for the cure and the control the various types of severe asthmatics.

3.2.1 Genetic Association

Studies have suggested that genetic factors such as bone morphogenetic protein receptor type II (BMPR II) or a functional polymorphism of glucocorticoid-induced transcript 1 (GLCCI1) can affect the responsiveness for corticosteroids in asthma [85–88]. However, to date, the information on genetic association with steroid resistance is relatively weak, and there is no evidence for the link between the polymorphisms or structural abnormalities in glucocorticoid receptor (GR) and steroid resistance in asthmatic patients, although a polymorphism of GRβ is associated with a reduced response to corticosteroids [89].

3.2.2 Functional Changes of GRs

The GR phosphorylation by several kinases is an important component for the reduction of GR function through altering its binding stability, translocation into nucleus, binding to DNA, and interaction with other proteins including transcription factors and molecular chaperones [90]. In fact, p38 MAPK and c-Jun N-terminal kinase (JNK) can phosphorylate serine 226 (Ser226) on GR, which leads to the inhibition of GR binding with glucocorticoid and is mostly observed in peripheral blood mononuclear cells (PBMCs) from asthmatics [91, 92]. MKP-1, an endogenous inhibitor of p38 MAPK and JNK signaling, is activated by corticosteroids. In alveolar macrophages from patients with severe asthma with the reduced level of MKP-1 expression as well as murine macrophages from *MKP1* gene knockout mice, the reduction of steroid responsiveness has been found [93, 94]. In addition, the levels of serine/threonine phosphatase protein phosphatase 2A (PP2A) which can dephosphorylate GR are reduced in PBMCs from patients with steroid resistance [95]. Several microbial origin stimuli such as Staphylococcal enterotoxin B can induce steroid resistance through GR phosphorylation and GR nuclear translocation [96, 97]. In addition, GR can be nitrosylated by NO donors, resulting in reduced binding affinity for corticosteroids [98]. As well known, patients with severe asthma produce high levels of NO, which nitrosylates the GR at HSP90 binding site, resulting in the decrease of the affinity of GR to glucocorticoid as well as HSP90 [99].

3.2.3 GR Isoform Identity and Expression

GRα predominates in most cell types, but other isoforms do arise as a consequence of alternative splicing, and the responsiveness to glucocorticoids can be modulated by the relative levels of the expression of each GR isoform [100]. GRβ has been known to act as a dominant-negative inhibitor [101–104]. Some inflammatory environment increases expression of GRβ in airway epithelial cells and various inflammatory cells [105, 106]. Moreover, TGF-β1, which is known to be associated with asthmatic airway remodeling, has been shown to reduce glucocorticoid responses, partly via decreased GRα expression [107].

3.2.4 Pro-inflammatory Transcription Factor Activation

Transcription factors NF-κB, STAT5, and AP-1 have been implicated in the occurrence of steroid resistance in inflammatory cells. Among them, AP-1 physically interacts with GR, thereby preventing its binding to GREs and other transcriptional factors [108, 109], supporting high levels of AP-1, phosphorylated JNK, and c-Fos observed in inflammatory cells from glucocorticoid-resistant asthmatics [109, 110]. NF-κB activation is correlated inversely with glucocorticoid responsiveness in patients with severe asthma [111]. In addition, activation of IRF-1 by IFNs or TNF-α may contribute to steroid resistance in airway smooth muscle cells [112].

3.2.5 Defective Histone Acetylation

In asthmatics, there is strong evidence connecting decreased HDAC2 activity with steroid resistance; molecular mechanisms for the decreases in HDAC2 expression/activity have been elucidated recently [113–115]. In particular, phosphoinositide 3-kinase (PI3K)-δ activated by oxidative stress may be due to cigarette smoking is implicated in the phosphorylation and inactivation of HDAC2 [116]. These findings suggest that oxidative stress and activation of PI3K-δ signaling might be important mechanisms for steroid resistance in bronchial asthma.

3.2.6 Immune Mechanisms

Despite little information on the direct relationship with steroid resistance in airway disorders, murine Th17 cells seem to be steroid resistant [117]. In addition, IL-17 increases the expression of GRβ in airway epithelial cells [105]. The decrease of the secretion of IL-10 in regulatory T cells has been reported in patients with steroid-resistant asthma [118, 119]. However, there is very scarce available information on immune mechanisms associated with steroid resistance to date.

3.3 Type 2 Inflammation

Molecular features of severe asthma have largely focused on the presence or extent of type 2 inflammatory responses, which involve the typical allergic inflammatory cytokines IL-4, IL-5, and IL-13. Of course, it is well known that all asthmatics from mild disease to severe one possess the type 2

inflammatory signature [120–123]; however, in mild asthmatics, the presence of a type 2 inflammatory process appears to be linked to early-onset and allergic disease, while in severe asthma, the relationship with allergy seems to be lower than that in mild asthma [124–126]. Despite these differences, new asthma treatments targeting Th2 cytokines or their receptors have been developed by many pharmaceutical agencies. These therapies have consistently blocked Th2 inflammation and associated structural changes in the airways of antigen-challenged animal models; however, few have been successful when moved to the clinic [127]. Interestingly, based on the gathering data from various cohort analyses, severe asthmatics appear to exhibit more favorable therapeutic efficacy than mild or total asthmatic patients when Type 2 or Th2 inflammation-targeting medicine is applied, showing that many cases of severe asthma involve cells of both the innate and adaptive immune systems, often in association with other immune pathways [128].

3.3.1 T Helper Type 2 (Th2) Cell-Dependent Inflammations

Under Th1/Th2 paradigm, the traditional asthma was accepted as an airway inflammatory disorder driven by Th2-predominant immune response of adaptive immune system. Since a type 2 or Th2 inflammation plays an important role in the pathogenesis in all types of asthma, GATA3 or STAT6, a transcription factor expressed in Th2 cells and linked to expression of Th2-specific cytokines such as IL-4, IL-5, and IL-13, has been established as an attractive target in the treatment of asthma associated with Th2 responses [129–133]. Thus, in severe asthma showing limited responses to corticosteroid therapy in suppressing Th2 cytokines, GATA3 or STAT6 inhibition appears to be an alternative therapeutic approach for severe asthma [134, 135]. Moreover, because Th2 cells have been recognized as an important part of the mechanisms underlying asthma, a Th2-high asthma has been defined by the use of genes expressed in airway epithelial brushings, consisting of a set of IL-13-inducible genes comprising *POSTN*, *CLCA1*, and *SERPINB2* [123, 136]. Interesting finding is that only about 50% of patients with mild-to-moderate asthma had a Th2-high asthma phenotype and they exhibit more severe asthmatic manifestations including airway eosinophilia which has led to drawn the concept of Th2-high and Th2-low endotypes. Subsequently, several recent studies have revealed that in Th2-high severe asthmatics showing increased levels of type 2 inflammatory biomarkers (i.e., eosinophilia, exhaled nitric oxide (FeNO), and periostin), IL-4/13 or IL-5-directed therapies have shown promising results in each specific subgroup [137–154]. In fact, anti-IL-5 therapy significantly attenuated asthma symptoms, reduced exacerbation, improved lung function, and showed sparing effect of oral corticosteroid in severe asthmatic patients with blood or sputum eosinophilia [143–146, 155]. In addition, in patients with modestly elevated levels of blood eosinophils, treatment with the anti-IL-4Rα antibody therapy maintained and even improved asthma control in moderate-to-severe asthma [138]. Interestingly, the IL-13 antibody was only modestly efficacious in the total patient cohort, but it markedly improved lung function in patients with high-serum periostin levels [137]. Altogether, substantial evidence now supports the presence of ongoing type 2 inflammation in severe asthma, which can be successfully targeted to improve outcome. Given that type 2 inflammation exists in total asthmatics with all severities including mild asthma and the corticosteroid resistance is not usually observed in mild asthmatics, in the pathogenesis of severe asthma, type 2 cytokines from Th2 cells seem to function with other cytokines and/or mediators to affect various target cells, including mast cells, eosinophils, epithelial cells, and airway smooth muscle cells, in which there are needs to be further investigated to define more specific mechanisms.

3.3.2 Innate Lymphoid Type 2 Cell-Associated Inflammation

In addition to Th2 cells, cells of the innate immune system, such as NKT cells, alternatively activated macrophages, eosinophils, and mast cells, can produce type 2 cytokines [156]. Above all, recently ILC2s have unveiled their roles in the pathogenesis of severe asthma producing significant amount of the type 2 cytokines, especially IL-5 and IL-13 under the influence of epithelial cell-derived cytokines TSLP, IL-25, IL-33, and prostaglandin D2 (PGD2) [157–161]. Since approximately 25% of patients with severe asthma do not display atopy, it is possible that there are other environmental triggers that induce a type 2 response without invoking a Th2 response. Actually, epithelial cells can release these cytokines by the stimulation of proteases from various pathogen-associated molecular patterns (PAMPs; i.e., viruses, bacteria, and allergens) [162–164]. More interestingly, an in vitro study has demonstrated that both cultured T cells and ILC2s secreted IL-5 and IL-13 under rhinovirus infection showing more potent capacity of Th2 cytokine secretion in ILC2s than T cells [165]. This finding provide the message that Th2 or type 2 inflammation is able to be induced powerfully without antigen/allergen specificity by the epithelial activation linked to type 2 cytokine production of ILC2s through their mediators TSLP, IL-25, and IL-33. While there are still debates on the measurement of ILC2 numbers in lung, severe asthmatics harbor greater numbers of activated ILC2s in airways as compared with milder asthmatics or healthy controls [20, 166]. The importance of ILC2 in the pathogenesis of severe asthma is also emphasized by many researchers and clinicians along with needs for future investigations to define the mechanisms of ILC2 activation and specific contributions to severe asthma for the novel therapeutic approach to severe asthma.

3.4 Non-type 2 Inflammation

As described above, approximately half of all asthmatic patients do not have evidence of type 2 inflammation [123, 167, 168]. "Type 2-low asthma" is currently defined as the "apparent" absence of type 2 cytokines and their downstream signatures. Non-type 2 patients generally have adult-onset disease, often in association with obesity, post-infectious, neutrophilic, and smoking-related factors, and are less likely to be atopic or allergic [120, 169–171]. With narrowing the scope, it is increasingly clear that severe asthma has also various phenotypes [172]. Actually, in some subjects with severe asthma, neutrophils, in addition to eosinophils, are important effector cells [60, 173–175]. Furthermore, non-Th2 cytokines such as IFN-γ, IL-8, IL-18, and IL-17 have been observed to be elevated in subjects with severe asthma [46, 176–178].

3.4.1 Inflammasome

In allergic airway inflammation, briefly, the innate immune system senses various allergens such as dust mites and molds via pattern recognition receptors (PRRs) including TLR, CLR, and/or NLRs. Several members of the cytosolic NLR family (NLRP1, NLRP3, and NLRC4) act as central components of the multiprotein inflammasome complex [179]. Inflammasomes are a group of protein complexes that recognize a diverse set of inflammation-inducing stimuli and that control production of important pro-inflammatory cytokines such as IL-1β and IL-18 [180]. Unlikely other NLR family members which have been activated by each specific stimulus, NLRP3 is activated by a large variety of signals, including PAMPs, DAMPs, and bacterial toxins [181–183]. More interestingly, studies have demonstrated that NLRP3 inflammasome activation is critical for the induction of allergic airway inflammation in bronchial asthma [184, 185], with increased understanding of how adaptive and innate immunity generate downstream pathology of allergic inflammation [186]. Furthermore, as for severe asthma, recent interesting studies have revealed that steroid-resistant neutrophilic asthmatic manifestations were significantly controlled by the NLRP3 inflammasome activation and the severe asthmatic symptoms were dramatically attenuated by the blockade of IL-1β [187, 188]. More supportively, very recent transcriptomic analysis with sputum from moderate-to-severe asthma revealed that non-Th2 phenotypes included two transcriptome-associated clusters (TACs); one cluster is characterized by IFN-γ, TNF-α, and inflammasome-associated genes, and the other cluster is represented by genes of metabolic pathways, ubiquitination, and mitochondrial function [189]. Taken together, emerging evidence has suggested that inflammasome, specifically NLRP3 inflammasome and its effector pro-inflammatory cytokines IL-1β and/or IL-18, plays a critical role in steroid-refractory severe asthma providing a very promising target for the control of severe asthma, especially non-eosinophilic type.

3.4.2 TNF-α

TNF-α contributes to neutrophilic inflammation and airway hyperresponsiveness in murine models [190]. An interesting study enrolled patients with corticosteroid-refractory severe asthma reported that a soluble TNF-α receptor inhibitor increased post-bronchodilator FEV1 and decreased bronchial hyperresponsiveness compared with placebo [191]. However, one subsequent double-blind, randomized, placebo-controlled trial confirmed there were only small improvements in asthma control and systemic inflammation after 12 weeks of etanercept therapy compared with placebo [192]. Similarly, a large-scaled clinical trial using a humanized monoclonal antibody for TNF-α, golimumab, in patients with severe refractory asthma to high-dose ICS/LABA treatment did not improve lung function or reduce acute exacerbations [193]. Moreover, it was associated with increases in systemic infections and cancer, which led this trial to premature termination [193]. Considering that TNF-α is a pro-inflammatory Th1 cytokine that induces activation of macrophages and neutrophilic inflammation which linked to severe asthmatic phenotypes, it can be hypothesized as a potential target for the control of severe asthma. However, until present time, substantial evidence has indicated that blockade of TNF-α is not recommended at least for the control of severe asthma despite its good pharmacologic effects on other chronic severe inflammation such as rheumatoid arthritis and that defining the role of TNF-α in the pathogenesis of severe asthma is needed.

3.4.3 Th17 Cell-Dependent Inflammation

Th17 cells are CD4 + T cells that express IL-17A, IL-17E, IL-17F, and IL-22 and are able to mediate neutrophil activation via the production of CXCL8 (IL-8) [194, 195]. In fact, IL-17A is one of the key players in eosinophilic as well as neutrophilic airway inflammation using animal models of asthma induced by toluene diisocyanate or ovalbumin [196, 197]. Additionally, a murine model of steroid-resistant neutrophilic asthma showed significant increases of IL-17A and murine IL-8 homolog KC in lung tissues [198]. Recent accumulating evidence has demonstrated that overexpression of IL-17A and IL-17F has been shown in lung tissue from patients with asthma, with expression levels correlating with asthma severity, especially in patients with neutrophilic corticosteroid-resistant disease [176]. Although there is little information on the direct relationship with steroid resistance in airway disorders, IL-17 increases the expression of GRβ in airway epithelial cells [105]. On the other hand, NF-κB, one of potent pro-inflammatory transcription factor linked to steroid resistance, is associated with IL-17A expression, and they interact cooperatively in severe asthma [22, 198]. Recently, a positive feedback relationship between endoplasmic reticulum stress (ER stress) and IL-17A has been suggested as one of mechanisms of the pathogenesis of severe asthma [22, 199]. Despite the favorable data from animal studies and the potential as the novel therapeutic target for the control of severe asthma, human clinical study has reported that brodalumab, a human anti-interleukin-17RA monoclonal antibody, had no effect on asthma control scores, symptom-free days, and FEV1 in patients with inadequately controlled moderate-to-severe asthma who were receiving ICS therapy. Moreover, a follow-up study focusing on high-reversibility subgroups was stopped due to a poor efficacy, and to date there is no further development of this antibody in asthma. In the future, the identification of the specific target subgroup of patients with severe asthma and the development of novel useful biomarkers to identify the well responded group are important tasks for the therapeutic application of IL-17-targeting agents to severe asthmatics.

3.4.4 Infection and IFN-γ

Th1 cells are differentiated from Th0 in the presence of IL-12, IL-18, and IFN-γ and secrete the signature cytokine IFN-γ [200, 201]. Although IFN-γ has been traditionally associated with the protective role against viral and bacterial infections, several studies have revealed that IFN-γ is implicated in the pathogenesis of severe asthma [202–204]. Moreover, severe asthmatics showed increased levels of IFN-γ-expressing cells in subepithelium compared with the levels of mild or moderate asthmatics [178].

The contribution of IFN-γ to the pathogenesis of severe asthma can potentially be related to several situations. IFN-γ is usually induced by various infections which are closely linked to severe asthma and acute exacerbation of asthma [205]. In fact, under infectious condition, the generation of intracellular messenger cyclic-di-GMP induces type I IFNs as well as Th1 and Th17 immune responses mixed with a low Th2 response [206]. Additionally, a mixed Th1 and Th17 immune response along with a low Th2 response induced by a combination of HDM allergen and cyclic-di-GMP in the airways of mice was detectable even in the presence of a high dose of CS, mimicking the CS-refractory immune response in severe asthmatics [134]. When IFN-γ knockout mice and wild-type mice were subjected to the same experimental protocol, increased airway hyperresponsiveness in wild-type mice was completely attenuated in IFN-γ knockout mice suggesting the pathogenic role of IFN-γ in the severe asthma [134].

Meanwhile, IL-18 is also known as IFN-γ-inducing factor. After binding to its receptors on

Th1 cells, IL-18 activates transcription factors such as NF-κB, subsequently inducing production of both Th1 and Th2 cytokines by Th1 cells [207]. Supportively, IFN-γ also synergizes with type 2 cytokines such as IL-13 to promote nitro-oxidative stress in airway epithelial cells [208]. Chronic asthma model using IL-18 deficient mice revealed low IFN-γ level in BAL fluids which lead to less airway inflammation and remodeling [209]. In addition, as described above IL-18 is one of effector cytokines produced by NLRP3 inflammasome which is closely associated with the development, of neutrophilic steroid-resistant asthma [187]. In the neutrophilic steroid-resistant asthma model, IFN-γ expression was also significantly increased in lung tissues of mice indicating the association of IFN-γ with innate immune response such as NLRP3 inflammasome activation participated in the induction and maintenance of severe asthma.

Another factor associated with IFN-γ is secretory leukocyte protease inhibitor (SLPI) with reverse correlation and is reported as a link between IFN-γ and airway hyperresponsiveness [134, 210]. Interestingly, SLPI deficiency can activate TGF-β, a representative fibrotic inducing factor and wound healing factor in living organisms [211]. Severe asthmatics showed increased IFN-γ expression in BAL cells with low levels of SLPI in airway cells [134]. Considering the important action of TGF-β in airway remodeling, inverse correlation between SLPI and TGF-β can be responsible for persistent airway hyperresponsiveness in high IFN-γ condition of severe asthma [212, 213]. Taken together, the IFN-γ signaling pathway appears to be associated with disease severity and phenotypes of severe asthma in many ways.

3.5 Subcellular Organelles

3.5.1 Endoplasmic Reticulum (ER)

The ER is a specialized organelle that plays a central role in the biosynthesis, correct protein folding, and posttranslational modifications of secretory and membrane proteins [214, 215].

When ER is stressed by some conditions such as increased demand in protein folding load in ER lumen, cells evolve an adaptive response called unfolded protein response (UPR). For the normal molecular transport, the secretory pathway and the ER-associated degradation (ERAD) pathway should keep their intact systems with working normally [215, 216]. Any perturbations of these conditions including failure of the ER's adaptive capacity can reduce the ability of ER to perform the normal physiologic roles, causing ER stress. ER stress causes accumulation of unfolded and/or misfolded proteins in ER, interferes with protein synthesis and secretion, induces reactive oxygen species (ROS) generation, and increases inflammation partly via NF-κB activation [217]. Recent studies have unveiled the role of ER stress in the pathogenesis of various pulmonary disorders, including asthma, chronic obstructive pulmonary disease (COPD), idiopathic pulmonary fibrosis, and acute lung injury [198, 218–220]. In particular, neutrophilic steroid-resistant severe asthma animal model induced by OVA and LPS sensitization and challenge exhibited the significant increases in ER stress markers, glucose-regulated protein 78 (GRP78), and CCAAT/enhancer-binding protein homologous protein (CHOP), as well as UPR-related proteins in lung tissues and BAL cells [198]. More intriguingly, an ER stress regulator, 4-phenylbutyric acid (4-PBA), effectively attenuated steroid-refractory asthmatic features including bronchial hyperresponsiveness and airway inflammation as well as increases in ER stress linked to NF-κB activation which induces various severe inflammatory/immune responses in the lung. In particular, 4-PBA dramatically reduced the increased expression of IL-17, whereas it further enhanced the increase in IL-10 levels, resulting in the attenuation of steroid-resistant asthmatic features. Moreover, the additional data using LPS-stimulated airway epithelial cells revealed a positive feedback interaction between IL-17 and ER stress [22]. Consistent with this contention, a recent study has demonstrated that ER stress inducer, tunicamycin, aggravates ER stress in mouse bronchial epithelial cells and increased expression of inflammation indicators such as

IL-6, IL-8, and TNF-α in lung tissues of neutrophilic severe asthmatic mice [221]. In addition to neutrophilic severe asthmatic phenotype, eosinophil-dominant severe asthma with fungal sensitization (SAFS) also showed the significant elevation of ER stress in mice [222]. In this study, fungal allergen (i.e., *Aspergillus fumigatus*)-inhaled mice showed typical asthmatic manifestations including eosinophilic airway inflammation and airway hyperresponsiveness which were not responded to treatment with oral steroid, while all asthmatic features and increased ER stress were very well controlled by the pharmacologic blockade of PI3K-δ activity, suggesting that PI3K-δ is linked to the modulation of ER stress in fungus-related severe asthmatic inflammation.

The double-stranded RNA (dsRNA)-activated serine/threonine kinase R (PKR) is well characterized as an essential component of the innate antiviral response. In view of the relation with ER stress, PKR phosphorylates e-IF2α, one of the branches for UPR, and, at the same time, ER stress activates PKR which stimulates various inflammatory signaling pathways [223, 224]. With these background, a recent interesting study showed that poly (I:C)-induced exacerbation of neutrophilic severe asthmatic mice was closely associated with PKR phosphorylation as well as increased ER stress in lung tissues including bronchial epithelial cells [224].

These observations suggest that ER stress plays a critical role in pathogenesis of various phenotypes of severe asthma including neutrophilic, eosinophilic, and infection-related types, supporting that the ER stress targeting strategy seems to be able to overcome the steroid resistance in severe asthma.

3.5.2 Mitochondrial Dysfunction

Mitochondria are dynamic double-membrane organelles and possess their own genome and proteome [225]. They are associated with the synthesis and catabolism of metabolites, generation and detoxification of ROS, apoptosis, regulation of cytoplasmic and mitochondrial matrix calcium, and generation of adenosine triphosphate (ATP) by oxidative phosphorylation [226]. In addition, recent evidence has uncovered that the roles of mitochondria as a direct inflammatory and immune controller are not worked only by metabolic dysfunction such as mitochondrial ROS but also by their abnormal dynamics (i.e., fusion and fission) [179, 227–229]. With these new concept of mitochondrial biological roles, mitochondrial abnormalities appear to be implicated in the pathogenesis of various pulmonary disorders such as lung cancer, chronic obstructive pulmonary disorders (COPD), asthma, cystic fibrosis, and so on [230]. Particularly, recent experimental data revealed that increased generation of mitochondria ROS and alteration of mitochondrial DNA induced steroid-resistant neutrophilic asthmatic features through the activation of NLRP3 inflammasome in the lung and that restoration of mitochondrial ROS levels using mitochondrial-specific ROS scavenger dramatically attenuated steroid-resistant airway hyperresponsiveness and inflammation in mice [187].

Although more future researches and studies are needed to support the role of mitochondria in the pathogenesis of severe asthma, considering the classic importance of oxidative stress including ROS in the pathogenesis of bronchial asthma and the development of steroid resistance and to date disappointing results with the effects of antioxidant supplementation in human studies for asthma, it is expected that mitochondria-related pathogenic mechanisms can be a key to solve the several obstacles on the way to cure severe asthma.

References

1. Chiappara G, Gagliardo R, Siena A, Bonsignore MR, Bousquet J, Bonsignore G, et al. Airway remodelling in the pathogenesis of asthma. Curr Opin Allergy Clin Immunol. 2001;1(1):85–93.
2. Al-Muhsen S, Johnson JR, Hamid Q. Remodeling in asthma. J Allergy Clin Immunol. 2011;128(3):451–62.
3. Cohen L, Xueping E, Tarsi J, Ramkumar T, Horiuchi TK, Cochran R, et al. Epithelial cell proliferation contributes to airway remodeling in severe asthma. Am J Respir Crit Care Med. 2007;176(2):138–45.

4. Gras D, Bourdin A, Vachier I, de Senneville L, Bonnans C, Chanez P. An ex vivo model of severe asthma using reconstituted human bronchial epithelium. J Allergy Clin Immunol. 2012;129(5):1259–66.
5. Xiao C, Puddicombe SM, Field S, Haywood J, Broughton-Head V, Puxeddu I, et al. Defective epithelial barrier function in asthma. J Allergy Clin Immunol. 2011;128(3):549–56.
6. Laitinen LA, Heino M, Laitinen A, Kava T, Haahtela T. Damage of the airway epithelium and bronchial reactivity in patients with asthma. Am Rev Respir Dis. 1985;131(4):599–606.
7. Jeffery PK, Wardlaw AJ, Nelson FC, Collins JV, Kay AB. Bronchial biopsies in asthma. An ultrastructural, quantitative study and correlation with hyperreactivity. Am Rev Respir Dis. 1989;140(6):1745–53.
8. Barbato A, Turato G, Baraldo S, Bazzan E, Calabrese F, Panizzolo C, et al. Epithelial damage and angiogenesis in the airways of children with asthma. Am J Respir Crit Care Med. 2006;174(9):975–81.
9. Holgate ST. Epithelium dysfunction in asthma. J Allergy Clin Immunol. 2007;120(6):1233–44.
10. Swartz MA, Tschumperlin DJ, Kamm RD, Drazen JM. Mechanical stress is communicated between different cell types to elicit matrix remodeling. Proc Natl Acad Sci U S A. 2001;98(11):6180–5.
11. Park JA, Tschumperlin DJ. Chronic intermittent mechanical stress increases MUC5AC protein expression. Am J Respir Cell Mol Biol. 2009;41(4):459–66.
12. Grainge CL, Lau LC, Ward JA, Dulay V, Lahiff G, Wilson S, et al. Effect of bronchoconstriction on airway remodeling in asthma. N Engl J Med. 2011;364(21):2006–15.
13. Park JA, Kim JH, Bi D, Mitchell JA, Qazvini NT, Tantisira K, et al. Unjamming and cell shape in the asthmatic airway epithelium. Nat Mater. 2015;14(10):1040–8.
14. Thomas B, Rutman A, Hirst RA, Haldar P, Wardlaw AJ, Bankart J, et al. Ciliary dysfunction and ultrastructural abnormalities are features of severe asthma. J Allergy Clin Immunol. 2010;126(4):722–9.
15. Locksley RM. Asthma and allergic inflammation. Cell. 2010;140(6):777–83.
16. Scanlon ST, AN MK. Type 2 innate lymphoid cells: new players in asthma and allergy. Curr Opin Immunol. 2012;24(6):707–12.
17. Bando JK, Nussbaum JC, Liang HE, Locksley RM. Type 2 innate lymphoid cells constitutively express arginase-I in the naive and inflamed lung. J Leukoc Biol. 2013;94(5):877–84.
18. Barlow JL, Peel S, Fox J, Panova V, Hardman CS, Camelo A, et al. IL-33 is more potent than IL-25 in provoking IL-13-producing nuocytes (type 2 innate lymphoid cells) and airway contraction. J Allergy Clin Immunol. 2013;132(4):933–41.
19. Nussbaum JC, Van Dyken SJ, von Moltke J, Cheng LE, Mohapatra A, Molofsky AB, et al. Type 2 innate lymphoid cells control eosinophil homeostasis. Nature. 2013;502(7470):245–8.
20. Smith SG, Chen R, Kjarsgaard M, Huang C, Oliveria JP, O'Byrne PM, et al. Increased numbers of activated group 2 innate lymphoid cells in the airways of patients with severe asthma and persistent airway eosinophilia. J Allergy Clin Immunol. 2016;137(1):75–86.
21. Siew LQ, Wu SY, Ying S, Corrigan CJ. Cigarette smoking increases bronchial mucosal IL-17A expression in asthmatics, which acts in concert with environmental aeroallergens to engender neutrophilic inflammation. Clin Exp Allergy. 2017;47(6):740–50.
22. Kim SR, Kim HJ, Kim DI, Lee KB, Park HJ, Jeong JS, et al. Blockade of interplay between IL-17A and endoplasmic reticulum stress attenuates LPS-induced lung injury. Theranostics. 2015;5(12):1343–62.
23. Gras D, Chanez P, Vachier I, Petit A, Bourdin A. Bronchial epithelium as a target for innovative treatments in asthma. Pharmacol Ther. 2013;140(3):290–305.
24. Pothoven KL, Norton JE, Suh LA, Carter RG, Harris KE, Biyasheva A, et al. Neutrophils are a major source of the epithelial barrier disrupting cytokine oncostatin M in patients with mucosal airways disease. J Allergy Clin Immunol. 2017;139(6):1966–78.
25. Levy BD, Bonnans C, Silverman ES, Palmer LJ, Marigowda G, Israel E. Diminished lipoxin biosynthe824sis in severe asthma. Am J Respir Crit Care Med. 2005;172(7):–30.
26. Bonnans C, Vachier I, Chavis C, Godard P, Bousquet J, Chanez P. Lipoxins are potential endogenous anti-inflammatory mediators in asthma. Am J Respir Crit Care Med. 2002;165(11):1531–5.
27. Ordoñez CL, Khashayar R, Wong HH, Ferrando R, Wu R, Hyde DM, et al. Mild and moderate asthma is associated with airway goblet cell hyperplasia and abnormalities in mucin gene expression. Am J Respir Crit Care Med. 2001;163(2):517–23.
28. Kuyper LM, Paré PD, Hogg JC, Lambert RK, Ionescu D, Woods R, et al. Characterization of airway plugging in fatal asthma. Am J Med. 2003;115(1):6–11.
29. Yu H, Li Q, Kolosov VP, Perelman JM, Zhou X. Interleukin-13 induces mucin 5AC production involving STAT6/SPDEF in human airway epithelial cells. Cell Commun Adhes. 2010;17(4–6):83–92.
30. Yan F, Li W, Zhou H, Wu Y, Ying S, Chen Z, et al. Interleukin-13-induced MUC5AC expression is regulated by a PI3K-NFAT3 pathway in mouse tracheal epithelial cells. Biochem Biophys Res Commun. 2014;446(1):49–53.
31. Nakano T, Inoue H, Fukuyama S, Matsumoto K, Matsumura M, Tsuda M, et al. Niflumic acid suppresses interleukin-13-induced asthma phenotypes. Am J Respir Crit Care Med. 2006;173(11):1216–21.
32. Benayoun L, Druilhe A, Dombret MC, Aubier M, Pretolani M. Airway structural alterations selec-

tively associated with severe asthma. Am J Respir Crit Care Med. 2003;167(10):1360–8.

33. Johnson PR, Roth M, Tamm M, Hughes M, Ge Q, King G, et al. Airway smooth muscle cell proliferation is increased in asthma. Am J Respir Crit Care Med. 2001;164(3):474–7.

34. Macedo P, Hew M, Torrego A, Jouneau S, Oates T, Durham A, et al. Inflammatory biomarkers in airways of patients with severe asthma compared with non-severe asthma. Clin Exp Allergy. 2009;39(11):1668–76.

35. Kaminska M, Foley S, Maghni K, Storness-Bliss C, Coxson H, Ghezzo H, et al. Airway remodeling in subjects with severe asthma with or without chronic persistent airflow obstruction. J Allergy Clin Immunol. 2009;124:45–51.

36. Tillie-Leblond I, de Blic J, Jaubert F, Wallaert B, Scheinmann P, Gosset P. Airway remodeling is correlated with obstruction in children with severe asthma. Allergy. 2008;63(5):533–41.

37. Woodruff PG, Dolganov GM, Ferrando RE, Donnelly S, Hays SR, Solberg OD, et al. Hyperplasia of smooth muscle in mild to moderate asthma without changes in cell size or gene expression. Am J Respir Crit Care Med. 2004;169:1001–6.

38. Kudo M, Melton AC, Chen C, Engler MB, Huang KE, Ren X, et al. IL-17A produced by T cells drives airway hyper-responsiveness in mice and enhances mouse and human airway smooth muscle contraction. Nat Med. 2012;18(4):547–54.

39. Goto K, Chiba Y, Sakai H, Misawa M. Tumor necrosis factor-alpha (TNF-alpha) induces upregulation of RhoA via NF-kappaB activation in cultured human bronchial smooth muscle cells. J Pharmacol Sci. 2009;110(4):437–44.

40. Chiba Y, Nakazawa S, Todoroki M, Shinozaki K, Sakai H, Misawa M. Interleukin-13 augments bronchial smooth muscle contractility with an upregulation of RhoA protein. Am J Respir Cell Mol Biol. 2009;40(2):159–67.

41. Ebina M, Takahashi T, Chiba T, Motomiya M. Cellular hypertrophy and hyperplasia of airway smooth muscles underlying bronchial asthma. A 3-D morphometric study. Am Rev Respir Dis. 1993;148(3):720–6.

42. Thomson RJ, Schellenberg RR. Increased amount of airway smooth muscle does not account for excessive bronchoconstriction in asthma. Can Respir J. 1998;5(1):61–2.

43. Jeffery PK. Remodeling in asthma and chronic obstructive pulmonary disease. Am J Respir Crit Care Med. 2001;164(10 Pt 2):S28–38.

44. Aubier M, Thabut G, Hamidi F, Guillou N, Brard J, Dombret MC, et al. Airway smooth muscle enlargement is associated with protease-activated receptor 2/ligand overexpression in patients with difficult-to-control severe asthma. J Allergy Clin Immunol. 2016;138(3):729–39.

45. Roche WR, Williams JH, Beasley R, Holgate ST. Subepithelial fibrosis in bronchi of asthmatics. Lancet. 1989;1(8637):520–4.

46. Chakir J, Shannon J, Molet S, Fukakusa M, Elias J, Laviolette M, et al. Airway remodeling-associated mediators in moderate to severe asthma: effect of steroids on TGF-beta, IL-11, IL-17, and type I and type III collagen expression. J Allergy Clin Immunol. 2003;111(6):1293–8.

47. Laitinen A, Altraja A, Kampe M, Linden M, Virtanen I, Laitinen LA. Tenascin is increased in airway basement membrane of asthmatics and decreased by an inhaled steroid. Am J Respir Crit Care Med. 1997;156(3 Pt 1):951–8.

48. de Medeiros MM, da Silva LF, dos Santos MA, Fernezlian S, Schrumpf JA, Roughley P, et al. Airway proteoglycans are differentially altered in fatal asthma. J Pathol. 2005;207(1):102–10.

49. Brightling CE, Bradding P, Symon FA, Holgate ST, Wardlaw AJ, Pavord ID. Mast cell infiltration of airway smooth muscle in asthma. N Engl J Med. 2002;346(22):1699–705.

50. Brightling CE, Symon FA, Holgate ST, Wardlaw AJ, Pavord ID, Bradding P. Interleukin-4 and -13 expression is co-localised to mast cells within the airway smooth muscle in asthma. Clin Exp Allergy. 2003;33(12):1711–6.

51. Carroll NG, Mutavdzic S, James AL. Increased mast cells and neutrophils in submucosal mucous glands and mucus plugging in patients with asthma. Thorax. 2002;57(8):677–82.

52. Carroll N, Carello S, Cooke C, James A. Airway structure and inflammatory cells in fatal attacks of asthma. Eur Respir J. 1996;9(4):709–15.

53. Brightling CE, Desai D, Siddiqui S. Severe asthma: a consequence of over exuberant repair? Clin Exp Allergy. 2009;39(11):1630–2.

54. Bourdin A, Neveu D, Vachier I, Paganin F, Godard P, Chanez P. Specificity of basement membrane thickening in severe asthma. J Allergy Clin Immunol. 2007;119(6):1367–74.

55. Saunders R, Siddiqui S, Kaur D, Doe C, Sutcliffe A, Hollins F, et al. Fibrocyte localization to the airway smooth muscle is a feature of asthma. J Allergy Clin Immunol. 2009;123(2):376–84.

56. Wang CH, Huang CD, Lin HC, Lee KY, Lin SM, Liu CY, et al. Increased circulating fibrocytes in asthma with chronic airflow obstruction. Am J Respir Crit Care Med. 2008;178(6):583–91.

57. Bousquet J, Jeffery PK, Busse WW, Johnson M, Vignola AM. Asthma. From bronchoconstriction to airways inflammation and remodeling. Am J Respir Crit Care Med. 2000;161(5):1720–45.

58. Kips JC, Pauwels RA. Airway wall remodelling: does it occur and what does it mean? Clin Exp Allergy. 1999;29(11):1457–66.

59. Payne DN, Rogers AV, Adelroth E, Bandi V, Guntupalli KK, Bush A, et al. Early thickening of the reticular basement membrane in children

with difficult asthma. Am J Respir Crit Care Med. 2003;167(1):78–82.

60. Wenzel SE, Schwartz LB, Langmack EL, Halliday JL, Trudeau JB, Gibbs RL, et al. Evidence that severe asthma can be divided pathologically into two inflammatory subtypes with distinct physiologic and clinical characteristics. Am J Respir Crit Care Med. 1999;160(3):1001–8.

61. Dolhnikoff M, da Silva LF, de Araujo BB, Gomes HA, Fernezlian S, Mulder A, et al. The outer wall of small airways is a major site of remodeling in fatal asthma. J Allergy Clin Immunol. 2009;123(5):1090–7.

62. Saglani S, Lui S, Ullmann N, Campbell GA, Sherburn RT, Mathie SA, et al. IL-33 promotes airway remodeling in pediatric patients with severe steroid-resistant asthma. J Allergy Clin Immunol. 2013;132(3):676–85.

63. Castanhinha S, Sherburn R, Walker S, Gupta A, Bossley CJ, Buckley J, et al. Pediatric severe asthma with fungal sensitization is mediated by steroid-resistant IL-33. J Allergy Clin Immunol. 2015;136(2):312–22.

64. Vrugt B, Wilson S, Bron A, Holgate ST, Djukanovic R, Aalbers R. Bronchial angiogenesis in severe glucocorticoid-dependent asthma. Eur Respir J. 2000;15(6):1014–21.

65. Charan NB, Baile EM, Pare PD. Bronchial vascular congestion and angiogenesis. Eur Respir J. 1997;10(5):1173–80.

66. Walters EH, Soltani A, Reid DW, Ward C. Vascular remodeling in asthma. Curr Opin Allergy Clin Immunol. 2008;8(1):39–43.

67. Abdel-Rahman AM, El-Sahrigy SA, Bakr SI. A comparative study of two angiogenic factors: vascular endothelial growth factor and angiogenin in induced sputum from asthmatic children in acute attack. Chest. 2006;129(2):266–71.

68. Bradding P, Holgate ST. Immunopathology and human mast cell cytokines. Crit Rev Oncol Hematol. 1999;31(2):119–33.

69. Long WM, Yerger LD, Martinez H, Codias E, Sprung CL, Abraham WM, et al. Modification of bronchial blood flow during allergic airway responses. J Appl Physiol. 1988;65(1):272–82.

70. Wanner A. Circulation of the airway mucosa. J Appl Physiol. 1989;67(3):917–25.

71. Webber SE, Salonen RO, Corfield DR, Widdicombe JG. Effects of non-neural mediators and allergen on tracheobronchial blood flow. Eur Respir J Suppl. 1990;12:638–43.

72. Barnes PJ. Pathophysiology of asthma. Br J Clin Pharmacol. 1996;42(1):3–10.

73. Gallagher SJ, Shank JA, Bochner BS, Wagner EM. Methods to track leukocyte and erythrocyte transit through the bronchial vasculature in sheep. J Immunol Methods. 2002;271(1–2):89–97.

74. Redington AE, Roche WR, Madden J, Frew AJ, Djukanovic R, Holgate ST, et al. Basic fibro-blast growth factor in asthma: measurement in bronchoalveolar lavage fluid basally and following allergen challenge. J Allergy Clin Immunol. 2001;107(2):384–7.

75. Chetta A, Zanini A, Foresi A, D'Ippolito R, Tipa A, Castagnaro A, et al. Vascular endothelial growth factor up-regulation and bronchial wall remodelling in asthma. Clin Exp Allergy. 2005;35(11):1437–42.

76. Feltis BN, Wignarajah D, Zheng L, Ward C, Reid D, Harding R, et al. Increased vascular endothelial growth factor and receptors: relationship to angiogenesis in asthma. Am J Respir Crit Care Med. 2006;173(11):1201–7.

77. Lee KY, Lee KS, Park SJ, Kim SR, Min KH, Choe YH, et al. Clinical significance of plasma and serum vascular endothelial growth factor in asthma. J Asthma. 2008;45(9):735–9.

78. Lee HY, Min KH, Lee SM, Lee JE, Rhee CK. Clinical significance of serum vascular endothelial growth factor in young male asthma patients. Korean J Intern Med. 2017;32(2):295–301.

79. Lee KS, Kim SR, Park SJ, Min KH, Lee KY, Choe YH, et al. Mast cells can mediate vascular permeability through regulation of the PI3K-HIF-1alpha-VEGF axis. Am J Respir Crit Care Med. 2008;178(8):787–97.

80. Lee KS, Park SJ, Kim SR, Min KH, Lee KY, Choe YH, et al. Inhibition of VEGF blocks TGF-beta1 production through a PI3K/Akt signalling pathway. Eur Respir J. 2008;31(3):523–31.

81. Park SJ, Lee KS, Lee SJ, Kim SR, Park SY, Jeon MS, et al. L-2-Oxothiazolidine-4-carboxylic acid or α-lipoic acid attenuates airway remodeling: involvement of nuclear factor-κB (NF-κB), nuclear factor erythroid 2p45-related factor-2 (Nrf2), and hypoxia-inducible factor (HIF). Int J Mol Sci. 2012;13(7):7915–37.

82. Marwick JA, Caramori G, Casolari P, Mazzoni F, Kirkham PA, Adcock IM, et al. A role for phosphoinositol 3-kinase δ in the impairment of glucocorticoid responsiveness in patients with chronic obstructive pulmonary disease. J Allergy Clin Immunol. 2010;125(5):1146–53.

83. Kim SR, Lee KS, Park HS, Park SJ, Min KH, Moon H, et al. HIF-1α inhibition ameliorates an allergic airway disease via VEGF suppression in bronchial epithelium. Eur J Immunol. 2010;40(10):2858–69.

84. Lee KS, Park SJ, Kim SR, Min KH, Jin SM, Puri KD, et al. Phosphoinositide 3-kinase-delta inhibitor reduces vascular permeability in a murine model of asthma. J Allergy Clin Immunol. 2006;118(2):403–9.

85. Carmichael J, Paterson IC, Diaz P, Crompton GK, Kay AB, Grant IW. Corticosteroid resistance in asthma. Br Med J. 1981;282(6274):1419–22.

86. Hakonarson H, Bjornsdottir US, Halapi E, Bradfield J, Zink F, Mouy M, et al. Profiling of genes expressed in peripheral blood mononuclear cells predicts glucocorticoid sensitivity in asthma patients. Proc Natl Acad Sci U S A. 2005;102(41):14789–94.

87. Donn R, Berry A, Stevens A, Farrow S, Betts J, Stevens R, et al. Use of gene expression profiling to identify a novel glucocorticoid sensitivity determining gene, BMPRII. FASEB J. 2007;21(2):402–14.

88. Tantisira KG, Lasky-Su J, Harada M, Murphy A, Litonjua AA, Himes BE, et al. Genomewide association between GLCCI1 and response to glucocorticoid therapy in asthma. N Engl J Med. 2011;365(13):1173–83.

89. van den Akker EL, Russcher H, van Rossum EF, Brinkmann AO, de Jong FH, Hokken A, et al. Glucocorticoid receptor polymorphism affects transrepression but not transactivation. J Clin Endocrinol Metab. 2006;91(7):2800–3.

90. Weigel NL, Moore NL. Steroid receptor phosphorylation: a key modulator of multiple receptor functions. Mol Endocrinol. 2007;21(10):2311–9.

91. Mercado N, Hakim A, Kobayashı Y, Meah S, Usmani OS, Chung KF, et al. Restoration of corticosteroid sensitivity by p38 mitogen activated protein kinase inhibition in peripheral blood mononuclear cells from severe asthma. PLoS One. 2012;7(7):e41582.

92. Ismaili N, Garabedian MJ. Modulation of glucocorticoid receptor function via phosphorylation. Ann N Y Acad Sci. 2004;1024:86–101.

93. Abraham SM, Lawrence T, Kleiman A, Warden P, Medghalchi M, Tuckermann J, et al. Antiinflammatory effects of dexamethasone are partly dependent on induction of dual specificity phosphatase 1. J Exp Med. 2006;203(8):1883–9.

94. Bhavsar P, Hew M, Khorasani N, Alfonso T, Barnes PJ, Adcock I, et al. Relative corticosteroid insensitivity of alveolar macrophages in severe asthma compared to non-severe asthma. Thorax. 2008;63(9):784–90.

95. Kobayashi Y, Mercado N, Barnes PJ, Ito K. Defects of protein phosphatase 2A causes corticosteroid insensitivity in severe asthma. PLoS One. 2011;6(12):e27627.

96. Li LB, Goleva E, Hall CF, Ou LS, Leung DY. Superantigen-induced corticosteroid resistance of human T cells occurs through activation of the mitogen-activated protein kinase kinase/extracellular signal-regulated kinase (MEK-ERK) pathway. J Allergy Clin Immunol. 2004;114(5):1059–69.

97. Li JJ, Wang W, Baines KJ, Bowden NA, Hansbro PM, Gibson PG, et al. IL-27/IFN-gamma induce MyD88-dependent steroid-resistant airway hyperresponsiveness by inhibiting glucocorticoid signaling in macrophages. J Immunol. 2010;185(7):4401–9.

98. Galigniana MD, Piwien-Pilipuk G, Assreuy J. Inhibition of glucocorticoid receptor binding by nitric oxide. Mol Pharmacol. 1999;55(2):317–23.

99. Barnes PJ, Adcock IM. Glucocorticoid resistance in inflammatory diseases. Lancet. 2009;373(9678):1905–17.

100. Oakley RH, Cidlowski JA. Cellular processing of the glucocorticoid receptor gene and protein: new mechanisms for generating tissue-specific actions of glucocorticoids. J Biol Chem. 2011;286(5):3177–84.

101. Leung DY, Hamid Q, Vottero A, Szefler SJ, Surs W, Minshall E, et al. Association of glucocorticoid insensitivity with increased expression of glucocorticoid receptor beta. J Exp Med. 1997;186(9):1567–74.

102. Oakley RH, Jewell CM, Yudt MR, Bofetiado DM, Cidlowski JA. The dominant negative activity of the human glucocorticoid receptor beta isoform. Specificity and mechanisms of action. J Biol Chem. 1999;274(39):27857–66.

103. Goleva E, Li LB, Eves PT, Strand MJ, Martin RJ, Leung DY. Increased glucocorticoid receptor beta alters steroid response in glucocorticoid-insensitive asthma. Am J Respir Crit Care Med. 2006;173(6):607–16.

104. DeRijk RH, Schaaf M, de Kloet ER. Glucocorticoid receptor variants: clinical implications. J Steroid Biochem Mol Biol. 2002;81(2):103–22.

105. Vazquez-Tello A, Semlali A, Chakir J, Martin JG, Leung DY, Eidelman DH, et al. Induction of glucocorticoid receptor-beta expression in epithelial cells of asthmatic airways by T-helper type 17 cytokines. Clin Exp Allergy. 2010;40(9):1312–22.

106. Webster JC, Oakley RH, Jewell CM, Cidlowski JA. Proinflammatory cytokines regulate human glucocorticoid receptor gene expression and lead to the accumulation of the dominant negative beta isoform: a mechanism for the generation of glucocorticoid resistance. Proc Natl Acad Sci U S A. 2001;98(12):6865–70.

107. Salem S, Harris T, Mok JS, Li MY, Keenan CR, Schuliga MJ, Stewart AG. Transforming growth factor-b impairs glucocorticoid activity in the A549 lung adenocarcinoma cell line. Br J Pharmacol. 2012;166(7):2036–48.

108. Adcock IM, Lane SJ, Brown CA, Lee TH, Barnes PJ. Abnormal glucocorticoid receptor/AP-1 interaction in steroid resistant asthma. J Exp Med. 1995;182(6):1951–8.

109. Loke TK, Mallett KH, Ratoff J, O'Connor BJ, Ying S, Meng Q, et al. Systemic glucocorticoid reduces bronchial mucosal activation of activator protein 1 components in glucocorticoid-sensitive but not glucocorticoid-resistant asthmatic patients. J Allergy Clin Immunol. 2006;118(2):368–75.

110. Lane SJ, Adcock IM, Richards D, Hawrylowicz C, Barnes PJ, Lee TH. Corticosteroid-resistant bronchial asthma is associated with increased c-fos expression in monocytes and T lymphocytes. J Clin Invest. 1998;102(12):2156–64.

111. Goleva E, Kisich KO, Leung DY. A role for STAT5 in the pathogenesis of IL-2-induced glucocorticoid resistance. J Immunol. 2002;169(10):5934–40.

112. Bhandare R, Damera G, Banerjee A, Flammer JR, Keslacy S, Rogatsky I, et al. Glucocorticoid receptor interacting protein-1 restores glucocorticoid responsiveness in steroid-resistant airway structural cells. Am J Respir Cell Mol Biol. 2010;42(1):9–15.

113. Barnes PJ. Reduced histone deacetylase in COPD: clinical implications. Chest. 2006;129(1):151–5.

114. Hew M, Bhavsar P, Torrego A, Meah S, Khorasani N, Barnes PJ, et al. Relative corticosteroid insensitivity of peripheral blood mononuclear cells in severe asthma. Am J Respir Crit Care Med. 2006;174(2):134–41.

115. Murahidy A, Ito M, Adcock IM, Barnes PJ, Ito K. Reduction is histone deacetylase expression and activity in smoking asthmatics: a mechanism of steroid resistance. Proc Am Thorac Soc. 2005;2:A889.

116. To Y, Ito K, Kizawa Y, Failla M, Ito M, Kusama T, et al. Targeting phosphoinositide-3-kinase-d with theophylline reverses corticosteroid insensitivity in COPD. Am J Respir Crit Care Med. 2010;182(7):897–904.

117. McKinley L, Alcorn JF, Peterson A, Dupont RB, Kapadia S, Logar A, et al. TH17 cells mediate steroid-resistant airway inflammation and airway hyperresponsiveness in mice. J Immunol. 2008;181(6):4089–97.

118. Hawrylowicz CM. Regulatory T cells and IL-10 in allergic inflammation. J Exp Med. 2005;202(11):1459–63.

119. Xystrakis E, Kusumakar S, Boswell S, Peek E, Urry Z, Richards DF, et al. Reversing the defective induction of IL-10-secreting regulatory T cells in glucocorticoid resistant asthma patients. J Clin Invest. 2006;116(1):146–55.

120. Wu W, Bleecker E, Moore W, Busse WW, Castro M, Chung KF, et al. Unsupervised phenotyping of Severe Asthma Research Program participants using expanded lung data. J Allergy Clin Immunol. 2014;133(5):1280–8.

121. Fajt ML, Gelhaus SL, Freeman B, Uvalle CE, Trudeau JB, Holguin F, et al. Prostaglandin D2 pathway upregulation: relation to asthma severity, control, and TH2 inflammation. J Allergy Clin Immunol. 2013;131(6):1504–12.

122. Modena BD, Tedrow JR, Milosevic J, Bleecker ER, Meyers DA, Wu W, et al. Gene expression in relation to exhaled nitric oxide identifies novel asthma phenotypes with unique biomolecular pathways. Am J Respir Crit Care Med. 2014;190(12):1363–72.

123. Woodruff PG, Modrek B, Choy DF, Jia G, Abbas AR, Ellwanger A, et al. T-helper type 2-driven inflammation defines major subphenotypes of asthma. Am J Respir Crit Care Med. 2009;180(5):388–95.

124. Moore WC, Bleecker ER, Curran-Everett D, Erzurum SC, Ameredes BT, Bacharier L, et al. Characterization of the severe asthma phenotype by the National Heart, Lung, and Blood Institute's Severe Asthma Research Program. J Allergy Clin Immunol. 2007;119(2):405–13.

125. European Network for Understanding Mechanisms of Severe Asthma (ENFUMOSA) Study Group. The ENFUMOSA cross-sectional European multicentre study of the clinical phenotype of chronic severe asthma. Eur Respir J. 2003;22(3):470–7.

126. Shaw DE, Sousa AR, Fowler SJ, Fleming LJ, Roberts G, Corfield J, et al. Clinical and inflammatory characteristics of the European U-BIOPRED adult severe asthma cohort. Eur Respir J. 2015;46(5):1308–21.

127. Holgate ST. Pathophysiology of asthma: what has our current understanding taught us about new therapeutic approaches? J Allergy Clin Immunol. 2011;128(3):495–505.

128. Ray A, Raundhal M, Oriss TB, Ray P, Wenzel SE. Current concepts of severe asthma. J Clin Invest. 2016;126(7):2394–403.

129. Zhang DH, Cohn L, Ray P, Bottomly K, Ray A. Transcription factor GATA-3 is differentially expressed in murine Th1 and Th2 cells and controls Th2-specific expression of the interleukin-5 gene. J Biol Chem. 1997;272(34):21597–603.

130. Zheng W, Flavell RA. The transcription factor GATA-3 is necessary and sufficient for Th2 cytokine gene expression in CD4 T cells. Cell. 1997;89(4):587–96.

131. Zhang DH, Yang L, Cohn L, Parkyn L, Homer R, Ray P, et al. Inhibition of allergic inflammation in a murine model of asthma by expression of a dominant-negative mutant of GATA-3. Immunity. 1999;11(4):473–82.

132. Nakamura Y, Ghaffar O, Olivenstein R, Taha RA, Soussi-Gounni A, Zhang DH, et al. Gene expression of the GATA-3 transcription factor is increased in atopic asthma. J Allergy Clin Immunol. 1999;103(2 Pt 1):215–22.

133. Zhu J, Min B, Hu-Li J, Watson CJ, Grinberg A, Wang Q, et al. Conditional deletion of Gata3 shows its essential function in T(H)1-T(H)2 responses. Nat Immunol. 2004;5(11):1157–65.

134. Raundhal M, Morse C, Khare A, Oriss TB, Milosevic J, Trudeau J, et al. High IFN-γ and low SLPI mark severe asthma in mice and humans. J Clin Invest. 2015;125(8):3037–50.

135. Chiba Y, Todoroki M, Nishida Y, Tanabe M, Misawa M. A novel STAT6 inhibitor AS1517499 ameliorates antigen-induced bronchial hypercontractility in mice. Am J Respir Cell Mol Biol. 2009;41(5):516–24.

136. Woodruff PG, Boushey HA, Dolganov GM, Barker CS, Yang YH, Donnelly S, et al. Genome-wide profiling identifies epithelial cell genes associated with asthma and with treatment response to corticosteroids. Proc Natl Acad Sci U S A. 2007;104(40):15858–63.

137. Corren J, Lemanske RF, Hanania NA, Korenblat PE, Parsey MV, Arron JR, et al. Lebrikizumab treatment in adults with asthma. N Engl J Med. 2011;365(12):1088–98.

138. Wenzel S, Ford L, Pearlman D, Spector S, Sher L, Skobieranda F, et al. Dupilumab in persistent asthma with elevated eosinophil levels. N Engl J Med. 2013;368(26):2455–66.

139. Wenzel S, Wilbraham D, Fuller R, Getz EB, Longphre M. Effect of an interleukin-4 variant on late phase asthmatic response to allergen challenge

in asthmatic patients: results of two phase 2a studies. Lancet. 2007;370(9596):1422–31.

140. Krug N, Hohlfeld JM, Kirsten AM, Kornmann O, Beeh KM, Kappeler D, et al. Allergen-induced asthmatic responses modified by a GATA3-specific DNAzyme. N Engl J Med. 2015;372(21):1987–95.

141. Hanania NA, Wenzel S, Rosén K, Hsieh HJ, Mosesova S, Choy DF, et al. Exploring the effects of omalizumab in allergic asthma: an analysis of biomarkers in the EXTRA study. Am J Respir Crit Care Med. 2013;187(8):804–11.

142. Flood-Page P, Swenson C, Faiferman I, Matthews J, Williams M, Brannick L, et al. A study to evaluate safety and efficacy of mepolizumab in patients with moderate persistent asthma. Am J Respir Crit Care Med. 2007;176(11):1062–71.

143. Haldar P, Brightling CE, Hargadon B, Gupta S, Monteiro W, Sousa A, et al. Mepolizumab and exacerbations of refractory eosinophilic asthma. N Engl J Med. 2009;360(10):973–84.

144. Bel EH, Wenzel SE, Thompson PJ, Prazma CM, Keene ON, Yancey SW, et al. Oral glucocorticoid-sparing effect of mepolizumab in eosinophilic asthma. N Engl J Med. 2014;371(13):1189–97.

145. Ortega HG, Liu MC, Pavord ID, Brusselle GG, FitzGerald JM, Chetta A, et al. Mepolizumab treatment in patients with severe eosinophilic asthma. N Engl J Med. 2014;371(13):1198–207.

146. Castro M, Wenzel SE, Bleecker ER, Pizzichini E, Kuna P, Busse WW, et al. Benralizumab, an anti-interleukin 5 receptor α monoclonal antibody, versus placebo for uncontrolled eosinophilic asthma: a phase 2b randomised dose-ranging study. Lancet Respir Med. 2014;2(11):879–90.

147. Pavord ID, Korn S, Howarth P, Bleecker ER, Buhl R, Keene ON, et al. Mepolizumab for severe eosinophilic asthma (DREAM): a multicentre, double-blind, placebo-controlled trial. Lancet. 2012;380(9842):651–9.

148. Nair P, Pizzichini MM, Kjarsgaard M, Inman MD, Efthimiadis A, Pizzichini E, et al. Mepolizumab for prednisone-dependent asthma with sputum eosinophilia. N Engl J Med. 2009;360(10):985–93.

149. Castro M, Mathur S, Hargreave F, Boulet LP, Xie F, Young J, et al. Reslizumab for poorly controlled, eosinophilic asthma: a randomized, placebo-controlled study. Am J Respir Crit Care Med. 2011;184(10):1125–32.

150. Piper E, Brightling C, Niven R, Oh C, Faggioni R, Poon K, et al. A phase II placebo-controlled study of tralokinumab in moderate-to-severe asthma. Eur Respir J. 2013;41(2):330–8.

151. Barnes N, Pavord I, Chuchalin A, Bell J, Hunter M, Lewis T, et al. A randomized, double-blind, placebo-controlled study of the CRTH2 antagonist OC000459 in moderate persistent asthma. Clin Exp Allergy. 2012;42(1):38–48.

152. Pettipher R, Hunter MG, Perkins CM, Collins LP, Lewis T, Baillet M, et al. Heightened response of

eosinophilic asthmatic patients to the CRTH2 antagonist OC000459. Allergy. 2014;69(9):1223–32.

153. Erpenbeck VJ, Popov TA, Miller SD, Weinstein SF, Spector S, Magnusson B, et al. QAW309 (fevipiprant) improves lung function and control of asthma symptoms in patients with more severe air flow limitation: a proof-of-concept study. Eur Respir J. 2015;46(suppl 59):PA2125.

154. Gauvreau GM, O'Byrne PM, Boulet LP, Wang Y, Cockcroft D, Bigler J, et al. Effects of an anti-TSLP antibody on allergen-induced asthmatic responses. N Engl J Med. 2014;370(22):2102–10.

155. Castro M, Zangrilli J, Wechsler ME, Bateman ED, Brusselle GG, Bardin P, et al. Reslizumab for inadequately controlled asthma with elevated blood eosinophil counts: results from two multicentre, parallel, double-blind, randomised, placebo-controlled, phase 3 trials. Lancet Respir Med. 2015;3(5):355–66.

156. Holtzman MJ, Byers DE, Alexander-Brett J, Wang X. The role of airway epithelial cells and innate immune cells in chronic respiratory disease. Nat Rev Immunol. 2014;14(10):686–98.

157. Bernink JH, Germar K, Spits H. The role of ILC2 in pathology of type 2 inflammatory diseases. Curr Opin Immunol. 2014;31:115–20.

158. Martinez-Gonzalez I, Steer CA, Takei F. Lung ILC2s link innate and adaptive responses in allergic inflammation. Trends Immunol. 2015;36(3):189–95.

159. Lloyd CM, Saglani S. Epithelial cytokines and pulmonary allergic inflammation. Curr Opin Immunol. 2015;34:52–8.

160. Chang JE, Doherty TA, Baum R, Broide D. Prostaglandin D2 regulates human type 2 innate lymphoid cell chemotaxis. J Allergy Clin Immunol. 2014;133(3):899–901.

161. Xue L, Salimi M, Panse I, Mjösberg JM, McKenzie AN, Spits H, et al. Prostaglandin D2 activates group 2 innate lymphoid cells through chemoattractant receptor-homologous molecule expressed on TH2 cells. J Allergy Clin Immunol. 2014;133(4):1184–94.

162. Halim TY, Krauss RH, Sun AC, Takei F. Lung natural helper cells are a critical source of Th2 cell-type cytokines in protease allergen-induced airway inflammation. Immunity. 2012;36(3):451–63.

163. Chustz RT, Nagarkar DR, Poposki JA, Favoreto S Jr, Avila PC, Schleimer RP, et al. Regulation and function of the IL-1 family cytokine IL-1F9 in human bronchial epithelial cells. Am J Respir Cell Mol Biol. 2011;45(1):145–53.

164. Hsu J, Lanza DC, Kennedy DW. Antimicrobial resistance in bacterial chronic sinusitis. Am J Rhinol. 1998;12(4):243–8.

165. Jackson DJ, Makrinioti H, Rana BM, Shamji BW, Trujillo-Torralbo MB, Footitt J, et al. IL-33-dependent type 2 inflammation during rhinovirus-induced asthma exacerbations in vivo. Am J Respir Crit Care Med. 2014;190(12):1373–82.

166. Nagakumar P, Denney L, Fleming L, Bush A, Lloyd CM, Saglani S. Type 2 innate lymphoid cells in

induced sputum from children with severe asthma. J Allergy Clin Immunol. 2016;137(2):624–6.

167. Dweik RA, Sorkness RL, Wenzel S, Hammel J, Curran-Everett D, Comhair SA, et al. National Heart, Lung, and Blood Institute Severe Asthma Research Program. Use of exhaled nitric oxide measurement to identify a reactive, at-risk phenotype among patients with asthma. Am J Respir Crit Care Med. 2010;181(10):1033–41.

168. McGrath KW, Icitovic N, Boushey HA, Lazarus SC, Sutherland ER, Chinchilli VM, et al. A large subgroup of mild-to-moderate asthma is persistently noneosinophilic. Am J Respir Crit Care Med. 2012;185(6):612–9.

169. Moore WC, Meyers DA, Wenzel SE, Teague WG, Li H, Li X, et al. National Heart, Lung, and Blood Institute's Severe Asthma Research Program. Identification of asthma phenotypes using cluster analysis in the Severe Asthma Research Program. Am J Respir Crit Care Med. 2010;181(4):315–23.

170. Miranda C, Busacker A, Balzar S, Trudeau J, Wenzel SE. Distinguishing severe asthma phenotypes: role of age at onset and eosinophilic inflammation. J Allergy Clin Immunol. 2004;113(1):101–8.

171. Dixon AE, Pratley RE, Forgione PM, Kaminsky DA, Whittaker-Leclair LA, Griffes LA, et al. Effects of obesity and bariatric surgery on airway hyperresponsiveness, asthma control, and inflammation. J Allergy Clin Immunol. 2011;128(3):508–15.

172. Poon AH, Eidelman DH, Martin JG, Laprise C, Hamid Q. Pathogenesis of severe asthma. Clin Exp Allergy. 2012;42(5):625–37.

173. Ordoñez CL, Shaughnessy TE, Matthay MA, Fahy JV. Increased neutrophil numbers and IL-8 levels in airway secretions in acute severe asthma: clinical and biologic significance. Am J Respir Crit Care Med. 2000;161(4 Pt 1):1185–90.

174. Shaw DE, Berry MA, Hargadon B, McKenna S, Shelley MJ, Green RH, et al. Association between neutrophilic airway inflammation and airflow limitation in adults with asthma. Chest. 2007;132(6):1871–5.

175. Woodruff PG, Khashayar R, Lazarus SC, Janson S, Avila P, Boushey HA, et al. Relationship between airway inflammation, hyperresponsiveness, and obstruction in asthma. J Allergy Clin Immunol. 2001;108(5):753–8.

176. Al-Ramli W, Préfontaine D, Chouiali F, Martin JG, Olivenstein R, Lemière C, et al. TH17-associated cytokines (IL-17A and IL-17F) in severe asthma. J Allergy Clin Immunol. 2009;123(5):1185–7.

177. Pepe C, Foley S, Shannon J, Lemiere C, Olivenstein R, Ernst P, Ludwig MS, Martin JG, Hamid Q. Differences in airway remodeling between subjects with severe and moderate asthma. J Allergy Clin Immunol. 2005;116(3):544–9.

178. Shannon J, Ernst P, Yamauchi Y, Olivenstein R, Lemiere C, Foley S, et al. Differences in airway cytokine profile in severe asthma compared to moderate asthma. Chest. 2008;133(2):420–6.

179. Nakahira K, Haspel JA, Rathinam VA, Lee SJ, Dolinay T, Lam HC, et al. Autophagy proteins regulate innate immune responses by inhibiting the release of mitochondrial DNA mediated by the NALP3 inflammasome. Nat Immunol. 2011;12(3):222–30.

180. Davis BK, Wen H, Ting JP. The inflammasome NLRs in immunity, inflammation, and associated diseases. Annu Rev Immunol. 2011;29:707–35.

181. Dostert C, Pétrilli V, Van Bruggen R, Steele C, Mossman BT, Tschopp J, et al. Innate immune activation through Nalp3 inflammasome sensing of asbestos and silica. Science. 2008;320(5876):674–7.

182. Pétrilli V, Papin S, Dostert C, Mayor A, Martinon F, Tschopp J, et al. Activation of the NALP3 inflammasome is triggered by low intracellular potassium concentration. Cell Death Differ. 2007;14(9):1583–9.

183. Martinon F, Pétrilli V, Mayor A, Tardivel A, Tschopp J. Gout-associated uric acid crystals activate the NALP3 inflammasome. Nature. 2006;440(7081):237–41.

184. Besnard AG, Guillou N, Tschopp J, Erard F, Couillin I, Iwakura Y, et al. NLRP3 inflammasome is required in murine asthma in the absence of aluminum adjuvant. Allergy. 2011;66(8):1047–57.

185. Kool M, Pétrilli V, De Smedt T, Rolaz A, Hammad H, van Nimwegen M, et al. Cutting edge: alum adjuvant stimulates inflammatory dendritic cells through activation of the NALP3 inflammasome. J Immunol. 2008;181(6):3755–9.

186. Gregory LG, Lloyd CM. Orchestrating house dust mite-associated allergy in the lung. Trends Immunol. 2011;32(9):402–11.

187. Kim SR, Kim DI, Kim SH, Lee H, Lee KS, Cho SH, et al. NLRP3 inflammasome activation by mitochondrial ROS in bronchial epithelial cells is required for allergic inflammation. Cell Death Dis. 2014;5:e1498.

188. Kim RY, Pinkerton JW, Essilfie AT, Robertson AA, Baines KJ, Brown AC, et al. Role for NLRP3 inflammasome-mediated, IL-1β -dependent responses in severe, steroid-resistant asthma. Am J Respir Crit Care Med. 2017;196(3):283-97.

189. Kuo CS, Pavlidis S, Loza M, Baribaud F, Rowe A, Pandis I, et al. T-helper cell type 2 (Th2) and non-Th2 molecular phenotypes of asthma using sputum transcriptomics in U-BIOPRED. Eur Respir J. 2017;49(2):pii:1602135. doi:10.1183/13993003.02135–2016.

190. Kips JC, Tavernier J, Pauwels RA. Tumor necrosis factor causes bronchial hyperresponsiveness in rats. Am Rev Respir Dis. 1992;145(2 Pt 1):332–6.

191. Berry MA, Hargadon B, Shelley M, Parker D, Shaw DE, Green RH, et al. Evidence of a role of tumor necrosis factor alpha in refractory asthma. N Engl J Med. 2006;354(7):697–708.

192. Morjaria JB, Chauhan AJ, Babu KS, Polosa R, Davies DE, Holgate ST. The role of a soluble TNFalpha receptor fusion protein (etanercept) in corticosteroid refractory asthma: a double blind, randomised, placebo controlled trial. Thorax. 2008;63(7):584–91.

193. Wenzel SE, Barnes PJ, Bleecker ER, Bousquet J, Busse W, Dahlén SE, et al. A randomized, double-blind, placebo-controlled study of tumor necrosis factor-alpha blockade in severe persistent asthma. Am J Respir Crit Care Med. 2009;179(7):549–58.

194. Roussel L, Houle F, Chan C, Yao Y, Bérubé J, Olivenstein R, et al. IL-17 promotes p38 MAPK dependent endothelial activation enhancing neutrophil recruitment to sites of inflammation. J Immunol. 2010;184(8):4531–7.

195. Halwani R, Al-Muhsen S, Hamid Q. T helper 17 cells in airway diseases: from laboratory bench to bedside. Chest. 2013;143(2):494–501.

196. Kim SR, Lee KS, Park SJ, Min KH, Lee KY, Choe YH, et al. PTEN down-regulates IL-17 expression in a murine model of toluene diisocyanate-induced airway disease. J Immunol. 2007;179(10):6820–9.

197. Park SJ, Lee KS, Kim SR, Min KH, Choe YH, Moon H, et al. Peroxisome proliferator-activated receptor gamma agonist down-regulates IL-17 expression in a murine model of allergic airway inflammation. J Immunol. 2009;183(5):3259–67.

198. Kim SR, Kim DI, Kang MR, Lee KS, Park SY, Jeong JS, et al. Endoplasmic reticulum stress influences bronchial asthma pathogenesis by modulating nuclear factor-κB activation. J Allergy Clin Immunol. 2013;132(6):1397–408.

199. Kim SR, Lee YC. Endoplasmic reticulum stress and the related signaling networks in severe asthma. Allergy Asthma Immunol Res. 2015;7(2):106–17.

200. Lazarevic V, Glimcher LH. T-bet in disease. Nat Immunol. 2011;12(7):597–606.

201. Schoenborn JR, Wilson CB. Regulation of interferon-gamma during innate and adaptive immune responses. Adv Immunol. 2007;96:41–101.

202. Yu M, Eckart MR, Morgan AA, Mukai K, Butte AJ, Tsai M, et al. Identification of an IFN-gamma/mast cell axis in a mouse model of chronic asthma. J Clin Invest. 2011;121(8):3133–43.

203. Yoshida M, Leigh R, Matsumoto K, Wattie J, Ellis R, O'Byrne PM, et al. Effect of interferon-gamma on allergic airway responses in interferon-gamma-deficient mice. Am J Respir Crit Care Med. 2002;166(4):451–6.

204. Yang M, Kumar RK, Foster PS. Pathogenesis of steroid-resistant airway hyperresponsiveness: interaction between IFN-gamma and TLR4/MyD88 pathways. J Immunol. 2009;182(8):5107–15.

205. Dahlberg PE, Busse WW. Is intrinsic asthma synonymous with infection? Clin Exp Allergy. 2009;39(9):1324–9.

206. Ebensen T, Schulze K, Riese P, Link C, Morr M, Guzman CA. The bacterial second messenger cyclic diGMP exhibits potent adjuvant properties. Vaccine. 2007;25(8):1464–9.

207. Nakanishi K, Tsutsui H, Yoshimoto T. Importance of IL-18-induced super Th1 cells for the development of allergic inflammation. Allergol Int. 2010;59(2):137–41.

208. Voraphani N, Gladwin MT, Contreras AU, Kaminski N, Tedrow JR, Milosevic J, et al. An airway epithelial iNOS-DUOX2-thyroid peroxidase metabolome drives Th1/Th2 nitrative stress in human severe asthma. Mucosal Immunol. 2014;7(5):1175–85.

209. Yamagata S, Tomita K, Sato R, Niwa A, Higashino H, Tohda Y. Interleukin-18-deficient mice exhibit diminished chronic inflammation and airway remodelling in ovalbumin-induced asthma model. Clin Exp Immunol. 2008;154(3):295–304.

210. Jin FY, Nathan C, Radzioch D, Ding A. Secretory leukocyte protease inhibitor: a macrophage product induced by and antagonistic to bacterial lipopolysaccharide. Cell. 1997;88(3):417–26.

211. Ashcroft GS, Lei K, Jin W, Longenecker G, Kulkarni AB, Greenwell-Wild T, Hale-Donze H. T al. Secretory leukocyte protease inhibitor mediates non-redundant functions necessary for normal wound healing. Nat Med. 2000;6(10):1147–53.

212. Makinde T, Murphy RF, Agrawal DK. The regulatory role of TGF-beta in airway remodeling in asthma. Immunol Cell Biol. 2007;85(5):348–56.

213. Cockcroft DW, Davis BE. Airway hyperresponsiveness as a determinant of the early asthmatic response to inhaled allergen. J Asthma. 2006;43(3):175–8.

214. van Anken E, Braakman I. Versatility of the endoplasmic reticulum protein folding factory. Crit Rev Biochem Mol Biol. 2005;40(4):191–228.

215. Ron D, Walter P. Signal integration in the endoplasmic reticulum unfolded protein response. Nat Rev Mol Cell Biol. 2007;8(7):519–29.

216. Kim I, Xu W, Reed JC. Cell death and endoplasmic reticulum stress: disease relevance and therapeutic opportunities. Nat Rev Drug Discov. 2008;7(12):1013–30.

217. Zhang K, Kaufman RJ. From endoplasmic reticulum stress to the inflammatory response. Nature. 2008;454(7203):455–62.

218. Malhotra D, Thimmulappa R, Vij N, Navas-Acien A, Sussan T, Merali S, et al. Heightened endoplasmic reticulum stress in the lungs of patients with chronic obstructive pulmonary disease: the role of Nrf2-regulated proteasomal activity. Am J Respir Crit Care Med. 2009;180(12):1196–207.

219. Korfei M, Ruppert C, Mahavadi P, Henneke I, Markart P, Koch M, et al. Epithelial endoplasmic reticulum stress and apoptosis in sporadic idiopathic pulmonary fibrosis. Am J Respir Crit Care Med. 2008;178(8):838–46.

220. Kim HJ, Jeong JS, Kim SR, Park SY, Chae HJ, Lee YC, et al. Inhibition of endoplasmic reticulum stress alleviates lipopolysaccharide-induced lung inflam-

mation through modulation of NF-κB/HIF-1α signaling pathway. Sci Rep. 2013;3:1142.

221. Guo Q, Li H, Liu J, Xu L, Yang L, Sun Z, et al. Tunicamycin aggravates endoplasmic reticulum stress and airway inflammation via PERK-ATF4-CHOP signaling in a murine model of neutrophilic asthma. J Asthma. 2017;54(2):125–33.

222. Lee KS, Jeong JS, Kim SR, Cho SH, Kolliputi N, Ko YH, et al. Phosphoinositide 3-kinase-δ regulates fungus-induced allergic lung inflammation through endoplasmic reticulum stress. Thorax. 2016;71(1):52–63.

223. Cabanski M, Steinmüller M, Marsh LM, Surdziel E, Seeger W, Lohmeyer J. PKR regulates TLR2/TLR4-dependent signaling in murine alveolar macrophages. Am J Respir Cell Mol Biol. 2008;38(1):26–31.

224. Kim SR, Lee YC, Kim DI, Park HJ. Effects of PKR inhibitor on poly (I:C)-induced exacerbation of severe asthma. Eur Respir J. 2016;48(suppl 60):PA1099.

225. Emelyanov VV. Mitochondrial connection to the origin of the eukaryotic cell. Eur J Biochem. 2003;270(8):1599–618.

226. Cloonan SM, Choi AM. Mitochondria: commanders of innate immunity and disease? Curr Opin Immunol. 2012;24(1):32–40.

227. Akundi RS, Huang Z, Eason J, Pandya JD, Zhi L, Cass WA, et al. Increased mitochondrial calcium sensitivity and abnormal expression of innate immunity genes precede dopaminergic defects in Pink1-deficient mice. PLoS One. 2011;6(1):e16038.

228. d'Avila JC, Santiago AP, Amâncio RT, Galina A, Oliveira MF, Bozza FA. Sepsis induces brain mitochondrial dysfunction. Crit Care Med. 2008;36(6):1925–32.

229. Archer SL. Mitochondrial dynamics–mitochondrial fission and fusion in human diseases. N Engl J Med. 2013;369(23):2236–51.

230. Aravamudan B, Thompson MA, Pabelick CM, Prakash YS. Mitochondria in lung diseases. Expert Rev Respir Med. 2013;7(6):631–46.

Part III

Diagnostic Approaches to Severe Asthma

Biomarkers in Severe Asthma

4

Wenjing Li and Mark C. Glaum

4.1 Diagnostic Significance of Pulmonary Function Testing in Severe Asthma

Pulmonary function testing (PFT) includes various components that are divided into categories based on the type of lung function they measure, including spirometry, lung volumes, diffusing capacity, blood gas assessment, and exercise challenge. Among them, spirometry is the most widely used for monitoring progression of lung disease and response to treatment.

In severe asthma, many physiologic abnormalities occur, including airflow limitation, increased airway resistance, loss of lung elastic recoil, increased gas trapping, and ventilation/perfusion mismatch [1–12]. In addition, patients with severe asthma tend to have more airway hyperresponsiveness than those with mild-to-moderate disease [10, 11, 13]. These abnormalities lead to characteristic changes in PFT measurements including decreases in forced expiratory volume at 1 s (FEV1), forced vital capacity (FVC), and peak expiratory flow rate

(PEF), increases in residual volume to total lung capacity ratio (RV/TLC), body plethysmography, and forced oscillation technique (FOT) [14–20]. Each of these abnormalities is associated with loss of asthma control [21].

According to ERS/ATS (European Respiratory Society/American Thoracic Society) guidelines [22], severe asthma is defined as asthma (patients aged ≥6 years) that requires ongoing treatment with guideline-based medications for GINA (Global Initiative for Asthma) steps 4–5 (high-dose ICS (inhaled corticosteroids) and LABA (long-acting β adrenoceptor agonists) or leukotriene modifier/theophylline) for the previous 1 year or systemic corticosteroids for 50% of the previous 1 year to maintain control or which remains uncontrolled despite this therapy. One of the main criteria of "uncontrolled asthma" is airflow limitation defined as FEV1 <80% predicted (pre-bronchodilator) in the presence of a reduced FEV1/FVC (less than 0.7) [22].

In the evaluation of severe asthma, clinicians must first rule out comorbid conditions that mimic or exacerbate asthma including laryngeal/pharyngeal reflux, chronic rhinosinusitis, vocal cord dysfunction syndrome, and other cardiopulmonary syndromes. After a thorough history and examination, spirometry should be performed with both expiratory and inspiratory flow/volume loops pre- and post-bronchodilator administration [23]. Assuming bronchodilators have been withheld prior to the start of the study, a post-bronchodilator improvement in the FEV1

W. Li
Department of Allergy, Tongji Hospital,
Wuhan, Hubei 430030, China

M.C. Glaum (✉)
Division of Allergy-Immunology, Department of
Internal Medicine, Morsani College of Medicine,
University of South Florida, Tampa, FL 33612, USA
e-mail: mglaum@health.usf.edu

© Springer Nature Singapore Pte Ltd. 2018
Y.C. Lee et al. (eds.), *Severe Asthma*, https://doi.org/10.1007/978-981-10-1998-2_4

of 12–15% and 200 ml confirms reversible airway obstruction. If there are inconsistencies among history, physical features, and spirometry, other pulmonary function tests may be considered including diffusing capacity and bronchoprovocation testing, such as methacholine or exercise challenges (only in patients with relatively preserved lung function). After the diagnosis of asthma is confirmed, clinicians should continually evaluate patients' severity and control status based on symptom control, frequency of exacerbations, pulmonary function, rescue medication requirement, and quality of life measurement according to guideline-based recommendations.

Severe asthma is considered to be a group of heterogeneous diseases caused by different triggers and pathophysiological mechanisms [24]. To better understand this heterogeneity and improve asthma management, efforts have been made to characterize asthma phenotypes. In the identification of phenotypes, spirometry is routinely performed to define important parameters such as pre- and post-bronchodilator FEV1, FVC, FEV1/FVC ratio, PEF variability, and methacholine PC20 (concentration producing a 20% fall of FEV1) to evaluate airway obstruction and potential reversibility in both adults and children [25–29]. Schatz et al. recommended FEV1 as a central parameter in defining phenotypes [30]. Moore et al. of the SARP generated an algorithm using three variables: (1) baseline pre-bronchodilator FEV1, (2) maximal "max" FEV1 (post-bronchodilator FEV1, after 6–8 puffs of albuterol), and (3) age of onset of asthma. Through this algorithm, 80% of study subjects were assigned to the appropriate cluster from milder asthma (Cluster 1) to more severe disease (Clusters 4 and 5) [26]. Recently, the concept of overlap of asthma and COPD (chronic obstructive pulmonary) has garnered much attention. GINA described this entity as asthma-COPD overlap syndrome (ACOS) and defined it as persistent airflow limitation with several features usually associated with asthma and several features usually associated with COPD [31]. These patients typically demonstrate incompletely reversible airflow limitation with less than 12%

reversibility of FEV1 post-bronchodilator along with FEV1 <80% predicted and FEV1/FVC% <0.7 [32].

In the evaluation of therapeutic response to asthma medications, spirometry is frequently used as an outcome measure. Most clinical trials examining the effectiveness of a biologic drug in asthma, including omalizumab, mepolizumab, reslizumab, and lebrikizumab, utilized spirometric parameters (mainly FEV1) as a key indicator of clinical effectiveness. In daily assessment of asthma control, the PEFR (peak expiratory flow rate) is widely used by patients at home as a surrogate measure of FEV1 [33]. GINA asthma treatment guidelines recommend that spirometry be performed before treatment, 3–6 months later, and then annually [34].

Among all spirometric parameters, the FEV1 is the most reproducible and well standardized [35], and it is considered the gold standard measurement of airflow obstruction [36]. However, FEV1 may not always correlate with symptoms, as some evidence suggests that FEV1 can be normal in symptomatic children with poorly controlled asthma [37–40], and these types of asthmatics may show no acute response to bronchodilator [41]. In children with normal pre- and post-bronchodilator FEV1, some propose that $FEF_{25-75}\%$ might better correlate with bronchodilator responsiveness [42]. Perez et al. showed that in adults with moderate-to-severe asthma without significant proximal airway obstruction (normal FEV1 and FEV1/FVC), treated with ICS and LABA, evidence of small-airway impairment could be found in more than half of the patients. In addition, they pointed out that routinely used lung function tests, including FEV1 and FEV1/FVC, can underestimate small-airway obstruction [43]. In heterogeneous populations, FEF_{25-75} (forced expiratory flow at 25–75% of forced vital capacity) showed no superiority in clinical decision-making when compared with FEV1, FVC, and FEV1/FVC ratio [44]. But, in asthmatic children with normal FEV1, reduced FEF_{25-75} had been associated with increased asthma severity, need for systemic corticosteroids, and more frequent exacerbations [45]. In asthmatic adults, reduction in FEF_{25-75} could identify a group of patients with more severe symptoms, greater healthcare utilization, and elevated biomarkers of airway inflammation that was independent of FEV1 and FEV1/FVC [46]. A French study showed that small-airway obstruction (assessed by FEF_{25-75}) might contribute to the long-term persistence of asthma, and small-airway obstruction predicted a subsequent risk for poor asthma outcomes that was independent of the large airways [47]. In another pediatric study, FEF_{75} (forced expiratory flow at 75% of forced vital capacity) was shown to be more sensitive than FEV1 and more sensitive in measuring small-airway obstruction as compared to FEF_{25-75} and FEF_{50} (forced expiratory flow at 50% of forced vital capacity) and might be another parameter worthy of consideration in the clinical management of childhood asthma [48].

Pulmonary function testing is an essential biomarker for the diagnosis and management of asthma. The FEV1 and FEV1/FVC ratio are recommended as "gold standard" measurements for diagnosis of obstructive lung disease by the National Lung Health Education Program (NLHEP), the National Heart Lung and Blood Institute (NHLBI), and the World Health Organization (WHO) [49]. Other spirometric parameters that measure small-airway obstruction have the potential to play a unique role in the diagnosis and management of certain phenotypes of asthma. Further study is needed to delineate the utility of these spirometric parameters as potential biomarkers of severe asthma.

4.2 Exhaled Breath Including FeNO

4.2.1 FeNO

Fractional exhaled nitric oxide (FeNO) is a noninvasive biomarker of allergic airway inflammation that is increasingly utilized in clinical practice. FeNO measurement is a simple and well-tolerated procedure that is easily obtainable even in children and in patients with severe airway obstruction. The utility of FeNO in the assessment of airway inflammation and the monitoring of responsiveness to ICS therapy is the subject of ongoing clinical studies.

Nitric oxide (NO) is a biological mediator in mammals, and it is produced by nitric oxide synthase (NOS) in a variety of cell types [50, 51]. NO plays multiple roles in asthma pathogenesis [52–55]. In response to pro-inflammatory stimuli, NOS levels are upregulated, resulting in increased NO production in lung tissue and in exhaled breath [56–59]. Thus, exhaled NO is regarded as an indirect marker for upregulation of allergic airway inflammation. In the 1990s, patients with asthma were found to have high FeNO in their exhaled breath [60–63], and FeNO levels in these patients were noted to decrease in response to treatment with corticosteroids [64]. In both pediatric and adult asthmatics, FeNO levels were found to correlate with eosinophilia in sputum [65, 66], bronchoalveolar lavage fluid [58, 67], and bronchial biopsies [60, 61]. Increased FeNO levels also correlated with the degree of eosinophilic airway inflammation in allergen-induced asthma exacerbations [68]. In addition, elevated FeNO levels have been correlated with several clinical markers of asthma control, including bronchodilator reversibility, β-agonist use, nocturnal symptoms [69], and the use of ICS [70].

Measurement of FeNO is widely used in the assessment of eosinophilic airway inflammation in asthma, and it is used to help predict the effectiveness of corticosteroid treatment [71]. According to WHO and ATS clinical practice guidelines, FeNO levels appear to be associated with eosinophilic airway inflammation; however, an increased FeNO can only provide supportive rather than conclusive evidence for an asthma diagnosis. Nonetheless, FeNO continues to be an attractive noninvasive outcome marker of eosinophilic airway inflammation in a variety of asthma clinical studies.

Increased FeNO may serve as a strong risk factor for new-onset asthma in children [72, 73], as it was associated with increased airway responsiveness [72] and increased likelihood for newly diagnosed asthma in this population [72, 73]. Among children, Chien et al. found that serum IL-17 and FeNO levels were significantly higher in mild-to-severe persistent asthmatics as compared to intermittent asthmatics or healthy controls ($P < 0.05$) [74]. Among elderly asthmatics, Kawamatawong et al. found that neither high total IgE, high FeNO, nor atopic status was associated with an increased risk of uncontrolled asthma [75]. They suggested that because of the heterogeneity of asthma, particularly severe asthma, Th2-mediated inflammation might not be the sole influence on asthma severity, especially in an elderly subpopulation [75]. Dweik et al. also found that FeNO levels are similar in adult patients with severe and non-severe asthma, but elevated FeNO levels may help to identify patients with more severe asthma phenotypes, including those with higher airway reactivity, greater airflow limitation, and more ICU admissions [76]. Amelink et al. identified a distinct severe adult-onset asthma phenotype (66% non-atopic), in which high FeNO levels and sputum eosinophils were associated with asthma severity, indicating this phenotype is nonatopic with persistent eosinophilic airway inflammation [77].

According to the WHO asthma clinical practice guidelines, severe uncontrolled asthma is comprised of three groups [78]: untreated severe asthma, difficult-to-treat severe asthma, and treatment-resistant severe asthma. Among them, difficult-to-treat severe asthma could be controlled with combined ICS/LABA asthma medications, while treatment-resistant severe asthma may need other treatment strategies, including targeted biologic therapies [78, 79]. Many studies have attempted to identify asthma phenotypes by FeNO levels. Some studies suggest that patients with treatment-resistant severe asthma have higher baseline FeNO levels than those with difficult-to-treat severe asthma [80, 81]. In contrast, others show no difference in FeNO levels between these two groups [82]. De Andrade et al. proposed that FeNO levels and spirometry are helpful to distinguish between treatment-resistant and difficult-to-treat severe asthma prior to any intervention [80]. In severe refractory asthma, FeNO levels were higher in patients with an eosinophilic phenotype compared to those with a non-eosinophilic phenotype [83]. Tseliou et al.

showed that in severe refractory asthma, FeNO threshold values distinguish those with predominant eosinophilia from those with neutrophilia and that FeNO levels were reduced in patients with predominant neutrophilia regardless of the concomitant presence of eosinophilia [84].

FeNO levels may serve as a predictor of loss of asthma control [85, 86] and as a risk for exacerbations [86, 87]. However, FeNO is not currently recommended as a tool to guide therapy in the management of asthma [22]. In children with asthma, FeNO levels were shown to change prior to moderate exacerbations [88]. One report suggests that monitoring of FeNO level may prevent the progression of the remodeling associated with refractory/severe asthma [89]. However, other studies report that FeNO-guided management provides no benefit to asthma control [90, 91]. One study that took atopy into account while using FeNO to guide management of asthma reported a reduction in the number of children with severe exacerbations, although this reduction may have been related to increased ICS use. Similarly, Peirsman et al. found that FeNO measurement may lead to diminished rates of asthma exacerbations when used to guide treatment through increased use of leukotriene receptor antagonists and increased ICS doses [92]. Nonetheless, it remains to be seen if FeNO-guided therapy is clearly beneficial for improving asthma control [93]. In adult patients, many studies show that FeNO is no better than pulmonary function testing as a predictor of asthma control [87, 94, 95]. Calhoun et al. found that biomarker-based or symptom-based adjustment of ICS was not superior to physician assessment-based adjustment of inhaled corticosteroids in measuring time to treatment failure [96]. Two large meta-analyses regarding FeNO-guided management drew different conclusions. Petsky et al. suggested that tailoring of asthma treatment based on FeNO levels failed to improve asthma outcomes in children and adults [97]. While Essat et al. found that while FeNO-guided management showed no statistically significant benefit in reducing severe asthma exacerbations or ICS use, it did produce a statistically significant reduction in asthma exacerbations of any severity [98].

Other smaller studies suggest promising results. Malerba et al. conducted an open-label study in 14 mild-to-moderate asthmatic patients, without a control group. The investigators found that if long-term sputum Eos and FeNO levels were used to titrate doses of ICS, asthma patients experienced improved long-term clinical stability without significant increases in the corticosteroid dose as compared to asthmatics on fixed ICS therapy [99]. Gibson et al. suggested that FeNO-guided management may not be suitable to maintain control in all asthmatic patients, but it may be useful in a select asthmatic population [100].

One of the most valuable clinical aspects of FeNO is the potential to differentiate patients with asthma-like symptoms from asthmatics most likely to benefit from ICS. In corticosteroid-responsive asthmatics, elevated FeNO levels decrease quickly after treatment with ICS [101, 102]. FeNO levels are affected by many factors including infection and smoking status. Despite this, measurement of FeNO tends to be highly reproducible in an individual with or without asthma [103–107], so sequential measurements may be important in determining trends. The rapid decrease in FeNO levels in response to ICS adds to its utility in monitoring adherence and response to therapy [108].

In recent years, the introduction of targeted biologic therapies for the treatment of asthma has peaked interest in finding noninvasive biomarkers of airway inflammation that might help guide treatment decisions. FeNO has been examined as a potential predictor of the effectiveness of anti-IgE (omalizumab) and anti-IL-5 and anti-IL-13 treatment. Hanania et al. showed that after 48 weeks of anti-IgE treatment, reductions in exacerbation rates were greater in subjects with elevated FeNO levels, indicating that these patients may achieve greater benefit from omalizumab [109]. Sorkness et al. found that FeNO level, along with blood eosinophil count and body mass index, can predict omalizumab response [110]. Moreover, elevated FeNO levels may be indicative of a positive response to anti-IL-13/IL-4 [111, 112].

In 2005, the ATS and the European Respiratory Society (ERS) published "Recommendations for Standardized Procedures for the Online and Offline Measurement of Exhaled Lower Respiratory Nitric Oxide and Nasal Nitric Oxide" [113]. This publication provided standardized recommendations for the measurement of FeNO as well as online and offline NO measurement, so that online measurements can be standardized for testing at multiple sites. These guidelines also suggested that FeNO should be expressed in parts per billion (ppb), as compared to nanoliters per liter [113].

Several studies demonstrate that there is considerable overlap between FeNO levels in healthy subjects and asthmatics [71, 114, 115]. In general, FeNO levels can be affected by several factors, including genetics, age (especially in children), sex, atopy, weight, height, smoking status, and a nitrate-rich diet [114, 116–125]. Many technical factors can also affect FeNO measurement, such as technique, exhalation flow rate, nasal NO contamination, the type of NO analyzer used [101], and anti-inflammatory medications. As a result, ATS guidelines in 2011 recommended specific cutoff points in patients with airway disease or respiratory symptoms instead of reference values derived from a "normal" population [71]. Documentation of the FeNO measurement should also include additional information including the date, time of the day, age, sex, ethnicity, height, smoking status, reason for the test, prior diagnoses, and whether or not the patient was using inhaled or oral corticosteroids at the time of testing. The format of the reporting should include the device used to make the measurement, the number of measurements made, and the flow rate (current FDA-approved devices use 50 ml/s flow rate) [71].

Due to multiple confounding factors that potentially influence FeNO measurement, the interpretation of FeNO levels should always be considered within the clinical context in which the measurement is being obtained [71]. Trends rather than absolute levels of FeNO combined with symptom scores may be a better indicator of asthma control [126].

According to ATS/ERS guidelines, low FeNO less than 25 ppb (<20 ppb in children) may indicate that eosinophilic inflammation and responsiveness to corticosteroids are less likely [71]. A symptomatic patient with low FeNO levels may suggest the presence of non-eosinophilic inflammation, neutrophilic asthma, cystic fibrosis, or nonpulmonary comorbid conditions such as GERD, cardiac disease, or laryngospasm. Low FeNO levels in an asymptomatic asthma patient may reflect appropriate dose and adherence ICS therapy. FeNO greater than 50 ppb (>35 ppb in children) in symptomatic patients may indicate eosinophilic airway inflammation resulting from atopic asthma, eosinophilic bronchitis, ACOS, or inadequate ICS dosing. In asymptomatic asthmatic patients, high levels of FeNO may indicate that caution be exercised with ICS dose reduction. The proper interpretation of FeNO levels can be complex, and measurement of this biomarker should be taken in context with other clinical observations.

FeNO possesses many characteristics that make it an attractive biomarker for allergic asthma. Obtaining a FeNO measurement is simple, noninvasive, and reproducible; moreover, FeNO levels respond quickly to ICS and other asthma therapies. As a biomarker, the utility of FeNO has been examined in predicting asthma onset, grading asthma severity, and monitoring responsiveness to ICS and biological therapies. However there still remain many unanswered questions as to the applicability of FeNO in other asthma phenotypes, and further study is needed to confirm a beneficial role in the management of severe asthma.

4.2.2 Exhaled Breath Condensate (EBC)

According to ATS/ERS guidelines, exhaled breath condensate (EBC) is strictly defined as exhaled samples collected by cooling the exhaled breath [127]. EBC contains mainly condensed water vapor (>99%) [128, 129], and a small fraction of the sample contains nonvolatile compounds. Those nonvolatile molecules include markers of oxidative stress (e.g., H_2O_2, 8-isoprostane, aldehydes, nitrite, and nitrate), markers of inflammation (e.g., prostanoids, leukotriene, and epoxides), cytokines (including Th2 cytokines), and many other biomarkers. All of the biomarkers noted above can be hydrophilic or hydrophobic [130]. These biomarkers may play an important role in aiding the understanding of asthma pathogenesis, diagnosis, management, and identification of new therapeutic targets.

ATS/ERS guidelines made many recommendations on the preferred methodology for EBC collection. During the EBC sampling process, the patient should be in the sitting position wearing a noseclip during normal tidal breathing. Collection time and temperature can vary depending on the study objective, but these parameters should be kept the same within any one study and should be precisely reported. The condensing device should incorporate certain essential components including an inert material on the collecting surface, a sufficient salivary trap, a mouth piece with separated inlet (as an inhalation port) and outlet (to direct exhaled breath toward the condensing apparatus), and a low-resistance flow path (without a filter) between the subject and the condensing chamber [127].

The EBC measurement can be affected by many factors, so the report should contain detailed methodology for sample collection including a description of the sampling device, the collecting surface material, the volume of the dead space (if possible), the duration and temperature of collection, breathing pattern, use of noseclip, route of inhalation, method, and duration of sample storage. Additionally, intra-assay and inter-assay variability of the technique and intra-subject variability should be reported. Lastly, details of subjects should contain information related to upper airway disease, smoking status, and medication history [127].

Immediately after collection, EBC samples should be frozen and stored at −70 °C. Samples should be stored in aliquots to avoid multiple freeze/thaw cycles. Every potential mediator possesses unique physiochemical characteristics, so measurement techniques will vary based on the mediator studied.

4.2.3 Exhaled Breath Temperature (EBT)

The role of EBT in the diagnosis and management of asthma remains controversial. Many studies suggest that EBT is elevated in uncontrolled asthmatics as compared to well-controlled asthmatics and healthy controls [131–133], especially during exacerbations [131]. Several studies showed that elevated EBT levels correlated to FeNO levels [134, 135] and sputum eosinophils [134]. Piacentini et al. found that elevated EBT related to MMP-9 levels [136]. This suggested that EBT may act as a marker of airway remodeling. However, other studies suggest that EBT is unrelated to FeNO levels [137, 138] or sputum eosinophil counts and therefore that EBT cannot be recommended as a reliable biomarker in the diagnosis and management of asthma [137–139]. Nonetheless, EBT is a simple, noninvasive, and consistently reproducible physiologic parameter [138, 140, 141]. Conflicting results related to the utility of EBT as an asthma biomarker may be due to varying experimental designs and lack of standardization. As such, further research is warranted to explore the utility of EBT measurements in asthma management.

4.2.4 pH

The acidity (pH) of EBC is thought to reflect airway acidification and thus may serve as a surrogate marker of airway acid-base status. EBC pH can be measured by commercial devices or homemade equipment [142]. The mean pH of healthy subjects is 7.7, with a normal range of 7.4–8.8 [143]. However, the detection and utility of EBC pH in the management of asthma remain controversial. According to ATS/ERS guidelines, deaeration (gas standardization) with a CO_2 free gas (e.g., argon) can be performed to improve the stability of pH values [127]. But Effros et al. suggested that EBC pH could be influenced by many factors including buffer capacities, dilution, and salivary contamination and that deaeration with argon is insufficient and unnecessary [144].

Some studies showed that pH values decrease significantly in asthma patients, especially during exacerbations [145–147], while others showed no differences between asthma patients and healthy subjects [148, 149]. Leung et al. suggested that EBC pH values could be influenced by severity of asthma [150], but Liu et al. found no significant differences between the EBC pH values of severe asthma, non-severe asthma, and control subjects [149]. Most studies suggested that EBC pH levels were unaffected by either ICS or systemic corticosteroids [147–149, 151, 152], while Hunt et al. and Antus et al. found that EBC pH values increased after corticosteroid therapy [145, 146]. EBC pH appears to have no relationship with other clinical variables such as FEV1 and symptoms scores. Studies evaluating the relationship between EBC pH and other biomarkers, such as FeNO, are also conflicting. Tomasiak-Lozowska et al. suggested that EBC pH values and FeNO are inversely correlated [153], while other groups found they are not correlated [146, 148, 150]. Studies evaluating relationships between EBC pH and 8-isoprostane showed similar conflicting results [150, 154]. Some groups proposed that a specific profile of airway biomarkers might help predict a particular pattern of airway inflammation. This profile of airway biomarkers typically combined EBC pH and other airway biomarkers to predict airway inflammation [153] and to diagnose childhood asthma [151]. In 2014, a larger study including 110 asthmatic children found serial EBC pH measurements had limited utility in the differential diagnosis, evaluation, and management of asthma. As a result, these authors recommended against using EBC pH as a biomarker in the long-term assessment of childhood asthma [147].

4.2.5 Biomarkers of Oxidative Stress

4.2.5.1 H_2O_2

In asthma, there is elevated airway expression of products of oxidative stress. EBC levels of oxidative stress-related biomarkers, such as hydrogen peroxide (H_2O_2), nitrite/nitrate, 8-isoprostane, and others, vary with asthma exacerbations, disease severity, and medication use.

Hydrogen peroxide (H_2O_2) is a reactive oxygen species (ROS), and it is considered a marker of oxidative stress. H_2O_2 is generated from multiple cellular sources including neutrophils and eosinophils [155, 156]. In both adult and pediatric asthmatics, EBC levels of H_2O_2 are significantly higher than that of healthy controls [157–163] regardless of asthma severity [160, 161]. During acute exacerbations, EBC H_2O_2 levels are significantly elevated [162]. While one group reported no association of EBC H_2O_2 levels with asthma exacerbations, the authors conceded that the discrepancy in their data may have to do with issues related to sample collection, storage, and analysis [164]. H_2O_2 is often used in combination with other biomarkers making interpretation more complex. Several studies suggested that EBC H_2O_2 levels were negatively correlated with lung function, especially FEV1% [158–161]. Two groups showed no correlation between EBC H_2O_2 and lung function [163, 165]. Conflicting results were also found when comparing EBC H_2O_2 levels with other clinical variables such as symptom scores and ACT scores, with two studies showing a positive correlation [160, 165] and one showing no correlation [163]. In two studies, FeNO appeared to be uncorrelated with EBC H_2O_2 levels [158, 165]. There is also conflicting data as to whether EBC H_2O_2 levels reflect clinical response to corticosteroid treatment in asthmatics. Jöbsis et al. found that ICS-naïve patients have significantly higher level of H_2O_2 than healthy controls, while ICS-treated patients do not [157]. In contrast, Trischler et al. found that there was no difference in EBC H_2O_2 levels between ICS-naïve and ICS-treated patients, as both groups had significantly higher EBC H_2O_2 levels than controls [165]. While Al Obaidi et al. suggested that after 4 weeks of ICS and salbutamol treatment, poorly controlled patients still had significantly higher levels of EBC H_2O_2 than stable asthmatics. As a result, the authors recommended that EBC H_2O_2 levels might act as a predictor of non-response to

steroid treatment [166]. Teng et al. did a meta-analysis about EBC H_2O_2's role in the assessment of disease severity, disease control, and response to corticosteroid treatment. They suggested that EBC H_2O_2 levels could be a promising biomarker in guiding asthma treatment [167]. Other authors differed, with Caffarelli et al. and Trischler et al. both suggesting that EBC H_2O_2 levels might not predict the occurrence of exacerbations [162, 168].

4.2.5.2 8-Isoprostane

8-Isoprostane is a prostaglandin (PG)-F2-like compound belonging to the class of F2 isoprostanes, and it is produced by free radical-catalyzed peroxidation of arachidonic acid [169]. EBC 8-isoprostane is considered to be an indicator of airway oxidative stress. With the exception of one study [170], several other groups have observed significantly higher levels of EBC 8-isoprostane in asthmatic patients as compared with healthy subjects [171–178]. In addition, the levels of EBC 8-isoprostane correlated positively with the severity of asthma [171, 173, 176, 177, 179, 180]. However, EBC 8-isoprostane does not seem to correlate with FeNO, pulmonary function, or asthma control parameters [172, 173, 175, 179–183]. The relationship between Cys-LTs and 8-isoprostane is controversial. Some studies showed no correlation [173, 180], while others showed significant correlation [174, 176, 181].

8-Isoprostane levels appear to be resistant or partially resistant to the effects of ICS or oral corticosteroids [171, 174, 183]. Sood et al. found that EBC 8-isoprostane levels did not change significantly after inhalation allergen or methacholine challenge within 23 h. As a result, the authors suggested that elevated EBC 8-isoprostane levels might represent a state of chronic airway oxidative stress and might not acutely change following bronchoprovocation [169]. Taken together, these studies suggest that EBC 8-isoprostane may be an important biomarker of airway oxidative stress and asthma severity, but not an indicator of asthma control.

4.2.5.3 Nitrite/Nitrate

Total nitrites/nitrates are the end products of nitric oxide metabolism, and these may serve as another biomarker of oxidative stress [184]. Some studies found EBC nitrites/nitrates to be significantly elevated in asthmatics as compared to healthy controls [153, 185–188]. In addition, other groups looked for co-expression of EBC FeNO and nitrites/nitrates. Some studies showed that the combination was significantly correlated with asthma [153, 189], while others did not [187, 188, 190]. Attempts to correlate combined expression of EBC FeNO and nitrites/nitrates with pulmonary function and asthma control parameters also revealed conflicting results [185, 188, 191, 192].

4.2.5.4 ADMA

Asymmetric dimethylarginine (ADMA), a biomarker related to oxidative stress, was found to be increased in the lungs of animals with allergic airway inflammation, and it was associated with airway hyperresponsiveness in these animals [193]. Carraro et al. found higher levels of ADMA in the EBC of children with asthma as compared to that of healthy subjects. However, inhaled corticosteroids had little effect on EBC ADMA concentrations [194].

4.2.6 Arachidonic Acid Metabolites

4.2.6.1 Prostanoids Prostaglandins, Prostacyclin, and Thromboxanes

Prostaglandins, prostacyclin, and thromboxane A2 (TXA2) are produced from arachidonic acid via the cyclooxygenase pathway [195]. In this cascade, TXA2 is rapidly converted to TXB2, which is chemically more stable and serves as a potent bronchoconstrictor [196]. No significant differences were found in EBC PGE2, PGD2, and TxB2 levels between asthmatic non-smokers and healthy subjects; however, elevated EBC PGE2 levels were found in asthmatic smokers [172, 173, 197].

4.2.6.2 Leukotrienes

Leukotrienes (LTs) are a family of lipid-derived mediators synthesized through an arachidonic acid 5-lipoxygenase pathway by inflammatory cells of the airways, particularly mast cells and eosinophils [198, 199]. They are well-studied inflammatory mediators and play an important role in asthmatic airway inflammation [200, 201]. LTs are categorized into cysteinyl leukotrienes (Cys-LTs, i.e., LTC_4, LTD_4, and LTE_4) and LTB_4. LTs have an important pathophysiological role in asthma [199, 202]. Cys-LTs can increase airway smooth muscle contraction, vascular permeability, and mucus secretion, and they inhibit mucociliary clearance [196, 199, 203]. Having no bronchoconstrictor effect, LTB4 still may contribute to airway obstruction by causing local edema and increasing mucus secretion [199]. EBC Cys-LTs and LTB4 concentrations are significantly higher in asthmatic patients than in healthy controls as shown by numerous studies [173, 197, 204–207], and their increased levels correlate with asthma severity [208]. EBC Cys-LTs levels appear to decrease significantly in asthmatics treated with either ICS or systemic corticosteroids as compared to pretreatment levels [173, 209, 210]. A few studies indicate that elevated levels of EBC Cys-LTs may correlate with EBC 8-isoprostane levels, suggesting a possible link between oxidative stress and airway inflammation [174, 176, 181].

4.2.7 Cytokines and Chemokines

Inflammatory and structural cells of the lungs produce different cytokines [211]. Many kinds of EBC interleukins were found at increased levels in asthmatics, including IL-4 [212–214], IL-5 [215], IL-6 [212, 213, 216], IL-8 [217], IL-10 [218], IL-17 [217], and IL-33 [219], while EBC interferon-γ was found at decreased levels [212].

EBC chemokines such as RANTES and eotaxin-1 (CCL11) were detected at significantly increased levels in asthmatics compared with healthy subjects [217, 220–223], and both chemokines were expressed at even higher levels in

EBC from unstable asthmatics as compared to those with stable asthma [220–222]. Therefore, elevated expression of both RANTES and CCL11 in EBC seems to correlate with asthma severity.

4.2.8 Other Molecules

Other molecules elevated in EBC of asthmatic patients compared to EBC of healthy controls include adenosine (degradation product of adenosine triphosphate) [224], formate (an indicator of increased catabolism of endogenous S-nitrosothiols) [225], MMP-9 (a marker of the inflammatory damage) [226], aldehydes (markers of oxidative stress, lipid peroxides which reflect oxidant-induced damage) [227], and high-sensitivity c-reactive protein (hs-CRP, a well-studied inflammatory mediator) [228].

EBC is a biological sample in which countless biomarkers may be identified. Many of the potential biomarkers identified in EBC are the same as those detectable in blood, urine, and the gases found in exhaled breath [229]. Since expression level of most of these biomarkers is quite low, detection is often limited by assay sensitivity. The study of new biomarkers for asthma may be facilitated by the use of novel molecular detection techniques including volatile organic compound (VOC) analysis using gas chromatography-mass spectrometry (GC-MF), proteomics [230, 231], metabolomics [232], and genomics [233].

Volatile organic compounds (VOCs) are produced in the airways and other parts of the body. Reactive oxygen species (ROS) produced as a result of inflammation promote the degradation of polyunsaturated fatty acids in lipid structures (e.g., epithelial cell membrane) and generate volatile hydrocarbons. Then, these VOCs are transported to the alveoli through the bloodstream, excreted in exhaled breath [234–236], and may then be measured. Among a wide range of VOCs, many were shown to have positive or negative association with asthma, including alkanes [237–239], aldehydes [238], ethane

[240], acetone [241], and isoprene. In one study, alkanes seemed to have the highest correlation with asthma [239]. Measurement of VOCs have been examined as a biomarker to indicate the presence of asthma [242, 243], and several studies have suggested a role for exhaled VOC assessment as a tool to predict asthma severity [241, 244–246].

Although EBC appears promising as a noninvasive diagnostic tool for assessment of airway inflammation, lack of standardized methodology and validated measurement techniques limit the current utility of EBC biomarkers in the assessment and management of asthma.

4.3 Blood

4.3.1 IgE

IgE mediates type I hypersensitivity reactions. After binding to high-affinity FcεR1 receptors on mast cells and basophils, cross-linking of IgE on the cell surface results in degranulation and immediate release of preformed mediators and de novo synthesis of non-preformed mediators including interleukins, cysteinyl leukotrienes, and chemokines. These mediators act locally to recruit and activate eosinophils and other leukocytes leading to chronic airway inflammation. Total IgE and allergen-specific IgE are blood-derived biomarkers of atopic status. The presence of allergen-specific IgE is a defining characteristic of the atopic asthma phenotype [247, 248], and high levels of total IgE suggest an increased risk of asthma [249].

Omalizumab is a humanized monoclonal antibody that binds free IgE. ERS and ATS 2014 guidelines recommend a therapeutic trial of omalizumab in both adults and children with severe allergic asthma who remain uncontrolled despite optimized medical therapy [22]. Recommended dosing schedules for omalizumab are based on weight and total IgE levels that should be between 30 and 700 IU/L. However, in most clinical trials, serum total IgE and allergen-specific IgE did not predict the response to omalizumab therapy [250, 251].

4.3.2 Blood Eosinophils

Although not as specific sputum eosinophils, peripheral blood eosinophilia is an important asthma biomarker that is associated with elevated type 2 cytokines in the airway [252, 253]. Blood eosinophil counts are correlated with asthma severity, increased risk for exacerbations, and worsened outcomes [254–257]. Peripheral blood eosinophil counts positively correlate with symptom scores [257] and airway hyperresponsiveness [258] but correlate negatively with FEV1 [257]. High blood eosinophil counts predict responsiveness to systemic corticosteroids [259, 260], anti-IL-5 therapy [261–266], and anti-IgE therapy [109, 267]. In many cases, blood eosinophil levels decrease in response to afore named treatments [261, 262, 264–266, 268, 269].

Eosinophils reside mainly in tissue, but when elevated in the blood, their presence may reflect generalized allergic inflammation. The definition of high blood eosinophils remains controversial; however, most studies define a high eosinophil count as ranging from >150 to >400 cells/ml. Factors affecting blood eosinophil counts can include allergen exposure, parasitic infections, and current systemic glucocorticoid therapy. Despite these potentially confounding factors, eosinophil counts do predict therapeutic response to several biologic treatments used for asthma, and as such, blood eosinophil counts likely serve as a surrogate biomarker of eosinophilic airway inflammation [270].

4.3.3 Periostin

Periostin is an extracellular matrix protein secreted by airway epithelial cells and lung fibroblasts largely in response to IL-4 and IL-13 [271–275]. Periostin mediates collagen synthesis and fibrinogenesis and activates transforming growth factor-beta (TGF-β) [272] and contributes to subepithelial thickening of the airways [271]. In addition, periostin may accelerate eosinophil migration and infiltration into the tissue [276]. Periostin is also considered as an important structural mediator in mesenchymal remodeling, and it plays a key role in balancing tissue adaption in response to insult/injury [277].

Jia et al. in the BOBCAT study (Bronchoscopic Exploratory Research Study of Biomarkers in Corticosteroid-Refractory Asthma) identified serum periostin as the best systemic biomarker of airway eosinophilia in severe, uncontrolled asthma. In this study, periostin was superior to blood eosinophils, IgE levels, YKL-40, and FeNO in predicting severe asthma. The authors suggested that periostin would be a preferred biomarker to use in patient selection for asthma therapeutics targeting Th2 inflammation [278]. Higher serum periostin levels were found to be an independent predictor for development of airflow limitation in asthmatic patients on ICS [279] and to be a good predictor of increased risk for asthma exacerbations [280]. Woodruff et al. found that high baseline expression of periostin was associated with an optimal clinical response to corticosteroids and that expression of periostin was steroid-responsive [273]. Lebrikizumab is a monoclonal antibody that blocks activity of IL-13. In studies examining the effectiveness of lebrikizumab in treating moderate-to-severe uncontrolled asthmatics, those with high baseline serum periostin levels demonstrated a greater improvement in the rate of asthma exacerbations and FEV1 compared with those with low serum periostin levels [280, 281]. Serum periostin may also predict the response to omalizumab treatment. In a study examining use of biomarkers in the EXTRA study (A Study of Omalizumab in Subjects with Moderate to Severe Persistent Asthma), subjects treated with omalizumab with high baseline levels of periostin demonstrated a greater reduction in exacerbation rates as compared to subjects with low serum periostin [109]. As compared to other potential serum-derived biomarkers for asthma, serum periostin possesses two major advantages. First, serum measurement of periostin seems to closely reflect local periostin levels in the tissues [282, 283], and second, serum periostin basal levels are readily detectable, thus providing a baseline reference point to compare relative changes in expression [284].

Periostin levels have also been examined in sputum and EBC [285, 286]. EBC periostin levels were found to be elevated in asthmatic patients as compared to healthy controls, and sputum periostin levels were associated with persistent airflow limitation and an eosinophilic inflammatory phenotype even in the setting of high-dose ICS therapy [285].

Further study is needed to validate and clarify the potential utility of periostin as a biomarker in severe asthma. In particular, efforts to establish cutoffs for high and low values will be important in establishing the utility of this biomarker in defining asthma phenotypes and selecting patients for emerging biologic therapies.

4.3.4 Other Biomarkers

Patil et al. measured serum levels of cytokines, chemokines, growth factors, adhesion molecules, and cytokine receptors in chronic asthmatics and analyzed their association with asthma control and quality of life. Results demonstrated that many cytokines and growth factors (excluding IFN-γ) were expressed at significantly higher levels in asthmatics as compared to non-asthmatic controls. Particularly, IL-3, IL-18, fibroblast growth factor, hepatocyte growth factor, and stem cell growth factor-β levels were elevated significantly in poorly controlled asthmatics as compared to those that were well controlled [287]. In another study, RANTES, a key chemotactic factor in allergic airway inflammation, was significantly increased in patients with severe asthma, and increased RANTES levels were positively associated with eosinophil count and total serum IgE level but negatively correlated to FEV1[288]. Recently, Chambers et al. found the existence of IL-17A[high] and IFN-γ[high] immunophenotypes in patients with corticosteroid-resistant asthma [289]. Ciprandi et al. showed that serum levels of IL-23 were increased among asthmatic children and negatively correlated with pulmonary function [290].

Galectins are a family of animal lectins with variable cellular and extracellular localization affecting a variety of cellular processes and biological activities. Of these, galectin-9 and galectin-3 were found to be relevant to asthma. Galectin-9 promotes recruitment of eosinophils and promotes Th2 dominance [291], but galectin-9 also binds IgE, thus promoting antiallergic effects and may prevent acute asthma exacerbations [292, 293]. Galectin-3 promotes multiple cellular activities including adhesion, growth, chemoattraction, differentiation, apoptosis, and cell cycle regulation. Galectin 3 may also have IgE binding activities [294–296]. Mauri et al. suggested that galectin-3 could be considered as a reliable biomarker to predict response to omalizumab therapy in severe asthmatics [297].

Other serum markers have been found to be elevated in the blood of asthmatics. These markers include C3 and C4 complement [298], chitinase-like protein YKL-40 [299, 300] and OX40, and its ligands [301]. Serum leptin levels and body mass index have also been associated with the severity of airway inflammation in childhood asthma [302].

In recent years, research has focused on new avenues of exploration including proteomics, genomics, and metabolomics in an attempt to identify relevant biomarkers in severe asthma. The goal of identifying new biomarkers is to help improve the diagnosis, phenotyping, and management of this chronic and sometimes debilitating disease. Among these biomarkers, attractive candidates include C7 complement protein, alpha-1-antitrypsin [303], gamma fibrinogen and its isoforms, C3 complement fragments [304], fibronectin [305], arginase, and syntaxin [306]. In addition, Verrills et al. identified another series of candidate biomarkers that includes a panel of four acute-phase proteins (ceruloplasmin, haptoglobin, hemopexin, and α2-macroglobulin) that may be able to discriminate among asthma, COPD, and normal controls [307]. However, further investigation is needed to clarify the relevance of these systemic biomarkers in various aspects of asthma.

4.4 Bronchial Specimens

4.4.1 Biomarkers in Induced Sputum

Induced sputum is a noninvasive and feasible procedure to perform in asthmatic adults and most children [308]. This technique is much less invasive than bronchoscopy with bronchoalveolar lavage (BAL) or bronchial brush/biopsy. Induced sputum is usually performed by inhalation of hypertonic saline in increasing concentrations (3%, 4% and 5%) via ultrasonic nebulizer. Prior to the procedure, a baseline FEV1 is performed then repeated after inhalation of each concentration of saline. If the FEV1 decreases by 15%, after inhalation of any of the saline concentrations, the procedure is halted [309]. Investigators have employed a variety of techniques to improve the quality of sputum samples and their staining characteristics [310–315]. Induced sputum consists of the cell phase (e.g., eosinophils and neutrophils) and the supernatant (e.g., cytokines and chemokines). Both phases can be used for diagnosis, phenotyping, and classification of asthma and for predicting exacerbations.

4.4.2   Sputum Eosinophil and Neutrophil Counts

Because asthma is a heterogeneous disease, a variety of inflammatory cell types can be recovered from the airways. Profiles of the inflammatory cellular infiltrate obtained by induced sputum, biopsies, and BAL can be categorized as pauci-granulocytic, eosinophilic, neutrophilic, and mixed [316, 317].

Sputum eosinophils are expressed as a percentage of inflammatory cells [318]. Based on reference values from healthy individuals, sputum eosinophilia is defined as an eosinophil percentage ≥3% [252, 313]. Elevated sputum eosinophil counts can be associated with gender (females > males) and atopy. [319]. In asthmatic patients, sputum eosinophil counts were significantly higher compared to those from healthy subjects. Sputum eosinophilia was associated with airway hyperresponsiveness [320], airway obstruction [321], and severe exacerbations [320, 322, 323] and inversely correlated with FEV1 [324]. In addition, sputum eosinophil counts are elevated following allergen challenge [312].

Sputum eosinophils can be used to gauge response to therapy. In several studies, sputum eosinophilia could predict a favorable response to glucocorticoid treatment [325–327]. Sputum eosinophil counts are reduced by both ICS and systemic corticosteroid treatment [328, 329], while withdrawal of glucocorticoid therapy leads to a rapid increase in the number of sputum eosinophils [321]. In asthmatics receiving ICS therapy, an increase in sputum eosinophils may be predictive of an asthma exacerbation [323, 330, 331]. Wenzel et al. found a group of severe asthmatics that demonstrated persistent eosinophilic inflammation despite corticosteroid treatment [316]. However, in most asthma phenotypes, sputum eosinophil counts still represent a key marker of steroid responsiveness during asthma exacerbations [97].

In addition to predicting clinical response to glucocorticoids, sputum eosinophilia may also predict pharmacologic response to biologic therapies. In studies examining the effectiveness of IL-5 blockade in asthma, patients with persistent sputum eosinophilia receiving drug demonstrated significant reduction in sputum eosinophils, decreased exacerbations, and improved lung function [263, 265, 266]. In contrast, asthmatics treated with mepolizumab not pre-selected for elevated sputum eosinophils showed little to no benefit in multiple measures of asthma control [332].

Neutrophils also play an important role in airway inflammation, particularly in certain asthma phenotypes. Moore et al. found that sputum neutrophilia, either alone or with concurrent sputum eosinophilia, was the most common inflammatory cell pattern in patient clusters with moderate-to-severe asthma [333]. Similar results supporting an important role for airway neutrophils in severe asthma were reported by Wenzel et al. using BAL and biopsy specimens [334]. Sputum neutrophil counts correlated with lung function, even in the setting of ICS therapy [324]. In other studies, sputum neutrophil counts were inversely associated with post-bronchodilator FEV1 in asthmatics, suggesting that neutrophilic inflammation may contribute to persistent airway obstruction [94, 335]. In one study, the combination of increased sputum eosinophils and neutrophils was found in asthmatic patients with the lowest lung function, worst asthma control, increased symptoms, and highest healthcare utilization [322].

In healthy subjects, neutrophils are the most abundant inflammatory cells in induced sputum [319]. Cigarette smoking, infection, ozone, and endotoxin are all factors that can increase sputum neutrophil counts [319]. Established cutoffs for defining sputum neutrophilia are less clear than that for sputum eosinophilia, but typical ranges vary from 40% to 76% [26, 319, 322, 336]. The mechanism for airway neutrophilia in asthma is not clear. The use of corticosteroids may contribute to neutrophilia by suppressing T2 inflammation, and even Th1 factors may play a role [337–339]. Th17 immunity might also be a cause for neutrophilia [339–342]. Hastie et al. found that significant statistical associations exist between sputum eosinophil and neutrophil counts and other biomarkers (including blood eosinophil counts, total serum IgE levels, FeNO values, and FEV1%). However, none of these biomarkers could predict sputum eosinophil and neutrophil levels in individual subjects across the spectrum of severe asthma. So, the authors suggest that the assessment of sputum eosinophils and neutrophils should not be replaced by those other non-invasive biomarkers for now [343]. The collection of sputum cell counts has not been standardized, and the technique of sputum induction and processing of specimens can be laborious and costly. ERS/ATS guidelines from 2014 on the definition, evaluation, and treatment of severe asthma suggested that, in adults, treatment should be primarily guided by clinical criteria and that sputum eosinophil counts should only be performed in experienced centers [22]. Measurement of sputum eosinophilia is recommended only as a supplemental outcome for study population characterization, clinical trials, and observational studies [252].

4.4.3 Other Biomarkers

Many cytokines, chemokines, and bioactive molecules are found at higher levels in sputum samples from patients with severe asthma as compared to non-asthmatic controls. Some of these compounds that show promise as potential biomarkers include eosinophil cationic proteins (ECP), eosinophil-derived neurotoxin (EDN), eotaxin, IL-4, IL-5, IL-8, IL-13, IL-17, TNF-α, IL-6, IL-12, granulocyte-macrophage colony-stimulating factor (GMCF), urokinase plasminogen activator, plasminogen activator inhibitor-1, purine nucleotides, growth factors, antioxidants, and mucins [278, 279, 344–348]. Also, neurokinin A levels have been shown to be significantly elevated during acute asthma exacerbations [349].

In addition, several important mediators found in the sputum supernatant of severe asthmatics are associated with the remodeling process, and these include pro-collagen synthesis peptides, matrix metalloproteinases (MMPs), tissue inhibitors of metalloproteinase (TIMP), and TGF-β [350]. Elevated sputum levels of these mediators in asthmatic patients are not influenced by ICS and may help to explain why ICS have no effect on preventing or reversing airway remodeling [351].

Sputum hydrogen sulfide levels have been suggested as a possible asthma biomarker as levels were negatively correlated with FEV1% (reversible with albuterol) and positively associated with increased sputum neutrophil counts. Saito et al. suggested that sputum hydrogen sulfate levels might serve as a useful biomarker of neutrophilic inflammation and chronic airflow obstruction [352].

In addition to cell and bioactive molecules, many other biomarkers have been measured in induced sputum. Brickey et al. used sputum cells to investigate inflammasome-related gene expression [353]. Alexis et al. investigated genetic responses and cell surface phenotype markers in asthmatic patients following exposure to inhaled irritants and found that phagocytosis was significantly decreased in sputum macrophages in asthmatics with high eosinophils as compared to those with normal eosinophils [354, 355]. Loughlin et al. measured hydration status of the airways using the percentage of solid content of sputum and suggested that there was a direct relationship between neutrophil inflammation and airway hydration status in stable asthmatics [356].

4.4.4 Bronchoalveolar Lavage, Bronchial Wash, and Bronchial Biopsy

Bronchoalveolar lavage (BAL) and bronchial wash can recover samples with cell phase and fluid phase components just as in the case of induced sputum. Those items detected in sputum can also be measured in lavage and bronchial wash. Along with bronchial biopsy, these techniques can be useful tools to monitor and assess airway inflammation and remodeling [357]. Some authors suggest that BAL alone cannot be considered as a surrogate for induced sputum, because induced sputum (and bronchial wash) sample central bronchial airways [358], while BAL mainly recovers cells and mediators from distal airways. Alexis et al. found that cells recovered from BAL display a more active inflammatory phenotype than cells recovered from sputum and blood from the same individual [359].

For now, BAL and biopsy have limited applicability as a source of asthma biomarkers because bronchoscopy is invasive and expensive and can only be performed by well-trained professionals in a hospital setting. Despite these limitations, valuable information regarding the nature of asthmatic airway inflammation has been obtained through the use of BAL. Goleva et al. recently showed that a subset of subjects with glucocorticoid-resistant asthma demonstrates airway expansion of specific gram-negative bacteria that trigger growth factor β-activated kinase 1/mitogen-activated protein kinase activation, thus promoting glucocorticoid resistance [360]. Esnault et al. identified 57 genes that were highly expressed by BAL eosinophils after in vivo allergen challenge. Expression of 41 of these genes had not been previously described in eosinophils, and each is a potentially new candidate to further study the contribution of eosinophils to airway biology [361]. Vargas et al. identified several corticosteroid resistance-related receptors (EGFR, EGR1, ESR2, PGR), transcription factors (MYC, JAK), cytokines (IL-8, IL-6, IL-1B), one chemokine (CXCL1), one kinase (SRC), and one cyclooxygenase (PTGS2) using a protein-protein interaction network [362]. Park et al. found that the ApoA1 protein level is decreased in the airways of mild-to-moderate persistent asthmatics as compared to healthy controls. Together with mouse data, they suggested ApoA1 to be a promising therapeutic target because of its ability to promote repair of defective epithelium in inflamed airways [363].

4.5 Others

In addition to exhaled breath, blood, and sputum, urine is another biological by-product that may contain potential biomarkers important in the investigation of airway inflammation. Examples of urine-derived biomarkers include leukotrienes, prostaglandins, eosinophil protein X, bromotyrosine, and others.

Leukotrienes play a central role in the pathogenesis of allergic asthma [199, 202]. Among leukotrienes, leukotriene E4 (LTE4) is the stable end product of LTC4, which is the dominant cysteinyl leukotriene (Cys-LT) in lung tissue [364]. LTE4 is excreted in the urine in measurable amounts, so urinary LTE4 is regarded as a marker for systemic production of Cys-LTs [365, 366].

Urinary LTE4 levels are increased in asthmatic patients as compared with healthy subjects, and elevated LTE4 levels are associated with disease severity, exacerbations, and aspirin and allergen challenges [367–369]. In recurrent episodic wheezing children, increased basal levels of LTE4 were observed only in those who were allergic; however, during exacerbations, increased urinary LTE4 levels were found in both atopic and nonatopic wheezers [370]. One study showed that children scored with a positive Asthma Predictive Index (API) had higher urinary LTE4 levels than those with negative API [371]. Chiu et al. found that urinary LTE4 levels appeared to be highly associated with IgE sensitization and related allergic airway diseases after age 2 [372]. Aspirin-intolerant asthmatic patients also had significantly higher urinary LTE4 levels than aspirin-tolerant asthmatics [373]. ICS do not appear to alter urinary LTE4 excretion [374]. Conversely, 5-lipoxygenase inhibitors significantly reduce urinary LTE4 levels by blocking Cys-LT metabolism

[375]. Smoking also affects arachidonic acid metabolite synthesis in asthmatics, as measured by urinary LTE4 and tetranor PGDM (an abundant urinary metabolite reflecting PGD2 biosynthesis) [376]. In children exposed to second-hand tobacco smoke, elevated urinary LTE4 levels are associated with susceptibility to severe asthma exacerbations [377].

Prostaglandin (PG) D2 is a major cyclooxygenase product released by activated mast cells. After antigen challenge, PGD2 can cause bronchoconstriction and vasodilation in the airways of asthmatic patients [378]. PGD2 is unstable and is metabolized to 9α, 11β-PGF2 in the human lung; then PGF2 is rapidly excreted in the urine [379]. Several studies showed that 9α, 11β-PGF2 levels are elevated in children with acute asthma, exercise-induced asthma, and asthmatic patients undergoing allergen or aspirin challenge [379, 380]. Urinary 9α, 11β-PGF2 levels were negatively correlated with lung function, and high-dose corticosteroid therapy might reduce 9α, 11β-β concentrations [381].

Eosinophils can release four basic eosinophil granule proteins, major basic protein, eosinophil cationic protein, eosinophil protein X (EPX), and eosinophil peroxidase. Among them, EPX (also known as eosinophil-derived neurotoxin (EDN)) is the only one that can be accurately measured in urine [382]. In childhood asthma, the urinary EPX (uEPX) concentrations are increased in children with either symptomatic or asymptomatic asthma compared to controls [383]. uEPX levels are elevated during exacerbations and correlate with the severity of attacks in asthmatic children [384]. Levels of uEPX are responsive to asthma therapy, as Severien et al. found that after 3 months of anti-inflammatory treatment, uEPX levels significantly decreased [367]. In addition, Nuijsink et al. found that uEPX is associated with FEV1 and induced sputum eosinophil percentage [385].

Bromotyrosine (BrTyr) is the end product of protein bromination that is excreted in urine, and this by-product can act as a biomarker for eosinophil-mediated oxidative pathways [101, 386–388]. Urinary BrTyr levels are significantly higher in patients with asthma, and elevated BrTyr levels are associated with exacerbations

and spirometric parameters of airway obstruction [388]. Cowan et al. found that BrTyr levels could predict patients' response to corticosteroids especially when combined with FeNO. However, the magnitude of decrease did not correlate with the degree of clinical response to ICS [101].

References

1. The ENFUMOSA. cross-sectional European multicentre study of the clinical phenotype of chronic severe asthma. European Network for Understanding Mechanisms of Severe Asthma. Eur Respir J. 2003;22(3):470–7.
2. Pride NB, Permutt S, Riley RL, Bromberger-Barnea B. Determinants of maximal expiratory flow from the lungs. J Appl Physiol. 1967;23(5):646–62.
3. Mead J, Turner JM, Macklem PT, Little JB. Significance of the relationship between lung recoil and maximum expiratory flow. J Appl Physiol. 1967;22(1):95–108.
4. Gelb AF, Zamel N. Unsuspected pseudophysiologic emphysema in chronic persistent asthma. Am J Respir Crit Care Med. 2000;162(5):1778–82.
5. Woolcock AJ, Read J. The static elastic properties of the lungs in asthma. Am Rev Respir Dis. 1968;98(5):788–94.
6. Gelb AF, Schein A, Nussbaum E, Shinar CM, Aelony Y, Aharonian H, et al. Risk factors for near-fatal asthma. Chest. 2004;126(4):1138–46.
7. Sorkness RL, Bleecker ER, Busse WW, Calhoun WJ, Castro M, Chung KF, et al. Lung function in adults with stable but severe asthma: air trapping and incomplete reversal of obstruction with bronchodilation. J Appl Physiol. 2008;104(2):394–403.
8. Perez T, Chanez P, Dusser D, Devillier P. Prevalence and reversibility of lung hyperinflation in adult asthmatics with poorly controlled disease or significant dyspnea. Allergy. 2016;71(1):108–14.
9. Gibbons WJ, Sharma A, Lougheed D, Macklem PT. Detection of excessive bronchoconstriction in asthma. Am J Respir Crit Care Med. 1996;153(2):582–9.
10. Chapman DG, Berend N, Horlyck KR, King GG, Salome CM. Does increased baseline ventilation heterogeneity following chest wall strapping predispose to airway hyperresponsiveness? J Appl Physiol. 2012;113(1):25–30.
11. Kaminsky DA, Daud A, Chapman DG. Relationship between the baseline alveolar volume-to-total lung capacity ratio and airway responsiveness. Respirology. 2014;19(7):1046–51.
12. Bourdin A, Paganin F, Prefaut C, Kieseler D, Godard P, Chanez P. Nitrogen washout slope in poorly controlled asthma. Allergy. 2006;61(1):85–9.

13. Porsbjerg C, Rasmussen L, Nolte H, Backer V. Association of airway hyperresponsiveness with reduced quality of life in patients with moderate to severe asthma. Ann Allergy Asthma Immunol. 2007;98(1):44–50.

14. Thamrin C, Nydegger R, Stern G, Chanez P, Wenzel SE, Watt RA, et al. Associations between fluctuations in lung function and asthma control in two populations with differing asthma severity. Thorax. 2011;66(12):1036–42.

15. Wenzel S. Physiologic and pathologic abnormalities in severe asthma. Clin Chest Med. 2006;27(1): 29–40. v

16. Shi Y, Aledia AS, Galant SP, George SC. Peripheral airway impairment measured by oscillometry predicts loss of asthma control in children. J Allergy Clin Immunol. 2013;131(3):718–23.

17. Lutchen KR, Jensen A, Atileh H, Kaczka DW, Israel E, Suki B, et al. Airway constriction pattern is a central component of asthma severity: the role of deep inspirations. Am J Respir Crit Care Med. 2001;164(2):207–15.

18. Bates JH, Irvin CG, Farre R, Hantos Z. Oscillation mechanics of the respiratory system. Compr Physiol. 2011;1(3):1233–72.

19. Sferrazza Papa GF, Pellegrino GM, Pellegrino R. Asthma and respiratory physiology: putting lung function into perspective. Respirology. 2014;19(7):960–9.

20. Alfieri V, Aiello M, Pisi R, Tzani P, Mariani E, Marangio E, et al. Small airway dysfunction is associated to excessive bronchoconstriction in asthmatic patients. Respir Res. 2014;15:86.

21. Kelly VJ, Sands SA, Harris RS, Venegas JG, Brown NJ, Stuart-Andrews CR, et al. Respiratory system reactance is an independent determinant of asthma control. J Appl Physiol. 2013;115(9):1360–9.

22. Chung KF, Wenzel SE, Brozek JL, Bush A, Castro M, Sterk PJ, et al. International ERS/ATS guidelines on definition, evaluation and treatment of severe asthma. Eur Respir J. 2014;43(2):343–73.

23. Standards for the diagnosis and care of patients with chronic obstructive pulmonary disease (COPD) and asthma. This official statement of the American Thoracic Society was adopted by the ATS Board of Directors, November 1986. Am Rev Respir Dis 1987;136(1):225–44.

24. A plea to abandon asthma as a disease concept. Lancet. 2006;368(9537):705.

25. Haldar P, Pavord ID, Shaw DE, Berry MA, Thomas M, Brightling CE, et al. Cluster analysis and clinical asthma phenotypes. Am J Respir Crit Care Med. 2008;178(3):218–24.

26. Moore WC, Meyers DA, Wenzel SE, Teague WG, Li H, Li X, et al. Identification of asthma phenotypes using cluster analysis in the Severe Asthma Research Program. Am J Respir Crit Care Med. 2010;181(4):315–23.

27. Fitzpatrick AM, Teague WG, Meyers DA, Peters SP, Li X, Li H, et al. Heterogeneity of severe asthma

in childhood: confirmation by cluster analysis of children in the National Institutes of Health/National Heart, Lung, and Blood Institute Severe Asthma Research Program. J Allergy Clin Immunol. 2011;127(2):382–9 e1-13.

28. Schatz M, Hsu JW, Zeiger RS, Chen W, Dorenbaum A, Chipps BE, et al. Phenotypes determined by cluster analysis in severe or difficult-to-treat asthma. J Allergy Clin Immunol. 2014;133(6):1549–56.

29. Konstantellou E, Papaioannou AI, Loukides S, Patentalakis G, Papaporfyriou A, Hillas G, et al. Persistent airflow obstruction in patients with asthma: characteristics of a distinct clinical phenotype. Respir Med. 2015;109(11):1404–9.

30. Schatz M, Rosenwasser L. The allergic asthma phenotype. J Allergy Clin Immunol Pract. 2014;2(6):645–8. quiz 9

31. (GINA) GIfA. Diagnosis of diseases of chronic airflow limitation: asthma, COPD and Asthma-COPD Overlap Syndrome (ACOS). Global Strategy for Asthma Management and Prevention; 2014.

32. Gibson PG, McDonald VM. Asthma-COPD overlap 2015: now we are six. Thorax. 2015;70(7):683–91.

33. Finkelstein JA, Lozano P, Shulruff R, Inui TS, Soumerai SB, Ng M, et al. Self-reported physician practices for children with asthma: are national guidelines followed? Pediatrics. 2000;106(4 Suppl):886–96.

34. (GINA) GIfA. Pocket guide for asthma management and prevention (A pocket guide for health professionals updated 2016); 2016.

35. Miller MR, Hankinson J, Brusasco V, Burgos F, Casaburi R, Coates A, et al. Standardisation of spirometry. Eur Respir J. 2005;26(2):319–38.

36. Expert panel Report 2: guidelines for the diagnosis and management of asthma (EPR-2 1997). NIH Publication No. 97-4051. Bethesda, MD: U.S. Department of Health and Human Services; National Institutes of Health; National Heart, Lung, and Blood Institutes; National Asthma Education and Prevention Program; 1997.

37. Bacharier LB, Strunk RC, Mauger D, White D, Lemanske RF Jr, Sorkness CA. Classifying asthma severity in children: mismatch between symptoms, medication use, and lung function. Am J Respir Crit Care Med. 2004;170(4):426–32.

38. Paull K, Covar R, Jain N, Gelfand EW, Spahn JD. Do NHLBI lung function criteria apply to children? A cross-sectional evaluation of childhood asthma at National Jewish Medical and Research Center, 1999-2002. Pediatr Pulmonol. 2005;39(4):311–7.

39. Strunk RC, Weiss ST, Yates KP, Tonascia J, Zeiger RS, Szefler SJ, et al. Mild to moderate asthma affects lung growth in children and adolescents. J Allergy Clin Immunol. 2006;118(5):1040–7.

40. Group TCAMPR. Long-term effects of budesonide or nedocromil in children with asthma. The Childhood Asthma Management Program Research Group. N Engl J Med. 2000;343(15):1054–63.

41. Fitzpatrick AM, Gaston BM, Erzurum SC, Teague WG, National Institutes of Health/National Heart L, Blood Institute Severe Asthma Research P. Features of severe asthma in school-age children: atopy and increased exhaled nitric oxide. J Allergy Clin Immunol. 2006;118(6):1218–25.

42. Simon MR, Chinchilli VM, Phillips BR, Sorkness CA, Lemanske RF Jr, Szefler SJ, et al. Forced expiratory flow between 25% and 75% of vital capacity and FEV1/forced vital capacity ratio in relation to clinical and physiological parameters in asthmatic children with normal FEV1 values. J Allergy Clin Immunol. 2010;126(3):527–34 e1-8.

43. Perez T, Chanez P, Dusser D, Devillier P. Small airway impairment in moderate to severe asthmatics without significant proximal airway obstruction. Respir Med. 2013;107(11):1667–74.

44. Quanjer PH, Weiner DJ, Pretto JJ, Brazzale DJ, Boros PW. Measurement of FEF25-75% and FEF75% does not contribute to clinical decision making. Eur Respir J. 2014;43(4):1051–8.

45. Rao DR, Gaffin JM, Baxi SN, Sheehan WJ, Hoffman EB, Phipatanakul W. The utility of forced expiratory flow between 25% and 75% of vital capacity in predicting childhood asthma morbidity and severity. J Asthma. 2012;49(6):586–92.

46. Riley CM, Wenzel SE, Castro M, Erzurum SC, Chung KF, Fitzpatrick AM, et al. Clinical implications of having reduced mid forced expiratory flow rates (FEF25-75), independently of FEV1, in adult patients with asthma. PLoS One. 2015;10(12):e0145476.

47. Siroux V, Boudier A, Dolgopoloff M, Chanoine S, Bousquet J, Gormand F, et al. Forced midexpiratory flow between 25% and 75% of forced vital capacity is associated with long-term persistence of asthma and poor asthma outcomes. J Allergy Clin Immunol. 2016;137(6):1709–16. e6

48. Francisco B, Ner Z, Ge B, Hewett J, Konig P. Sensitivity of different spirometric tests for detecting airway obstruction in childhood asthma. J Asthma. 2015;52(5):505–11.

49. Mottram C. Ruppel's manual of pulmonary function testing. 10th ed. Amsterdam: Elsevier; 2012.

50. Ignarro LJ, Buga GM, Wood KS, Byrns RE, Chaudhuri G. Endothelium-derived relaxing factor produced and released from artery and vein is nitric oxide. Proc Natl Acad Sci U S A. 1987;84(24):9265–9.

51. Palmer RM, Ashton DS, Moncada S. Vascular endothelial cells synthesize nitric oxide from L-arginine. Nature. 1988;333(6174):664 6.

52. Dweik RA, Comhair SA, Gaston B, Thunnissen FB, Farver C, Thomassen MJ, et al. NO chemical events in the human airway during the immediate and late antigen-induced asthmatic response. Proc Natl Acad Sci U S A. 2001;98(5):2622–7.

53. Ricciardolo FL. Multiple roles of nitric oxide in the airways. Thorax. 2003;58(2):175–82.

54. Khatri SB, Hammel J, Kavuru MS, Erzurum SC, Dweik RA. Temporal association of nitric oxide levels and airflow in asthma after whole lung allergen challenge. J Appl Physiol. 2003;95(1):436–40. discussion 5

55. Khatri SB, Ozkan M, McCarthy K, Laskowski D, Hammel J, Dweik RA, et al. Alterations in exhaled gas profile during allergen-induced asthmatic response. Am J Respir Crit Care Med. 2001;164(10 Pt 1):1844–8.

56. Guo FH, De Raeve HR, Rice TW, Stuehr DJ, Thunnissen FB, Erzurum SC. Continuous nitric oxide synthesis by inducible nitric oxide synthase in normal human airway epithelium in vivo. Proc Natl Acad Sci U S A. 1995;92(17):7809–13.

57. Guo FH, Erzurum SC. Characterization of inducible nitric oxide synthase expression in human airway epithelium. Environ Health Perspect. 1998;106(Suppl 5):1119–24.

58. Guo FH, Uetani K, Haque SJ, Williams BR, Dweik RA, Thunnissen FB, et al. Interferon gamma and interleukin 4 stimulate prolonged expression of inducible nitric oxide synthase in human airway epithelium through synthesis of soluble mediators. J Clin Invest. 1997;100(4):829–38.

59. Guo FH, Comhair SA, Zheng S, Dweik RA, Eissa NT, Thomassen MJ, et al. Molecular mechanisms of increased nitric oxide (NO) in asthma: evidence for transcriptional and post-translational regulation of NO synthesis. J Immunol. 2000;164(11):5970–80.

60. Alving K, Weitzberg E, Lundberg JM. Increased amount of nitric oxide in exhaled air of asthmatics. Eur Respir J. 1993;6(9):1368–70.

61. Kharitonov SA, Yates D, Robbins RA, Logan-Sinclair R, Shinebourne EA, Barnes PJ. Increased nitric oxide in exhaled air of asthmatic patients. Lancet. 1994;343(8890):133–5.

62. Gaston B, Drazen J, Chee CBE, Wohl MEB, Stamler JS. Expired nitric oxide concentrations are elevated in patients with reactive airways disease. Endothelium. 1993;1:87–92.

63. Jouaville LF, Annesi-Maesano I, Nguyen LT, Bocage AS, Bedu M, Caillaud D. Interrelationships among asthma, atopy, rhinitis and exhaled nitric oxide in a population-based sample of children. Clin Exp Allergy. 2003;33(11):1506–11.

64. Silkoff PE, McClean P, Spino M, Erlich L, Slutsky AS, Zamel N. Dose-response relationship and reproducibility of the fall in exhaled nitric oxide after inhaled beclomethasone dipropionate therapy in asthma patients. Chest. 2001;119(5):1322–8.

65. Dweik RA, Erzurum SC. Regulation of nitric oxide (NO) synthases and gas phase NO by oxygen. In: Marczin N, Kharitonov SA, Yacoub MH, Barnes PJ, editors. Disease markers in exhaled breath (lung biology in health and disease). New York: Marcel Dekker, Inc; 2003. p. 235–46.

66. Hansel TT, Kharitonov SA, Donnelly LE, Erin EM, Currie MG, Moore WM, et al. A selective inhibitor of inducible nitric oxide synthase inhibits exhaled

breath nitric oxide in healthy volunteers and asthmatics. FASEB J. 2003;17(10):1298–300.

67. Gustafsson LE, Leone AM, Persson MG, Wiklund NP, Moncada S. Endogenous nitric oxide is present in the exhaled air of rabbits, guinea pigs and humans. Biochem Biophys Res Commun. 1991;181(2):852–7.

68. Ricciardolo FL, Di Stefano A, Silvestri M, Van Schadewijk AM, Malerba M, Hiemstra PS, et al. Exhaled nitric oxide is related to bronchial eosinophilia and airway hyperresponsiveness to bradykinin in allergen-induced asthma exacerbation. Int J Immunopathol Pharmacol. 2012;25(1):175–82.

69. Covar RA, Szefler SJ, Martin RJ, Sundstrom DA, Silkoff PE, Murphy J, et al. Relations between exhaled nitric oxide and measures of disease activity among children with mild-to-moderate asthma. J Pediatr. 2003;142(5):469–75.

70. Smith AD, Cowan JO, Taylor DR. Exhaled nitric oxide levels in asthma: personal best versus reference values. J Allergy Clin Immunol. 2009;124(4):714–8. e4

71. Dweik RA, Boggs PB, Erzurum SC, Irvin CG, Leigh MW, Lundberg JO, et al. An official ATS clinical practice guideline: interpretation of exhaled nitric oxide levels (FENO) for clinical applications. Am J Respir Crit Care Med. 2011;184(5):602–15.

72. Kotaniemi-Syrjanen A, Malmberg LP, Malmstrom K, Pelkonen AS, Makela MJ. Factors associated with elevated exhaled nitric oxide fraction in infants with recurrent respiratory symptoms. Eur Respir J. 2013;41(1):189–94.

73. Singer F, Luchsinger I, Inci D, Knauer N, Latzin P, Wildhaber JH, et al. Exhaled nitric oxide in symptomatic children at preschool age predicts later asthma. Allergy. 2013;68(4):531–8.

74. Chien JW, Lin CY, Yang KD, Lin CH, Kao JK, Tsai YG. Increased IL-17A secreting CD4+ T cells, serum IL-17 levels and exhaled nitric oxide are correlated with childhood asthma severity. Clin Exp Allergy. 2013;43(9):1018–26.

75. Kawamatawong T, Siripongpun S, Rerkpattanapipat T. Role of eosinophilic inflammation and atopy in elderly asthmatic patients. Asia Pac Allergy. 2016;6(3):181–6.

76. Dweik RA, Sorkness RL, Wenzel S, Hammel J, Curran-Everett D, Comhair SA, et al. Use of exhaled nitric oxide measurement to identify a reactive, at-risk phenotype among patients with asthma. Am J Respir Crit Care Med. 2010;181(10):1033–41.

77. Amelink M, de Groot JC, de Nijs SB, Lutter R, Zwinderman AH, Sterk PJ, et al. Severe adult-onset asthma: a distinct phenotype. J Allergy Clin Immunol. 2013;132(2):336–41.

78. Bousquet J, Mantzouranis E, Cruz AA, Ait-Khaled N, Baena-Cagnani CE, Bleecker ER, et al. Uniform definition of asthma severity, control, and exacerbations: document presented for the World Health Organization Consultation on Severe Asthma. J Allergy Clin Immunol. 2010;126(5):926–38.

79. Lodrup Carlsen KC, Hedlin G, Bush A, Wennergren G, de Benedictis FM, De Jongste JC, et al. Assessment of problematic severe asthma in children. Eur Respir J. 2011;37(2):432–40.

80. de Andrade WC, Lasmar LM, Ricci Cde A, Camargos PA, Cruz AA. Phenotypes of severe asthma among children and adolescents in Brazil: a prospective study. BMC Pulm Med. 2015;15:36.

81. Sharples J, Gupta A, Fleming L, Bossley CJ, Bracken-King M, Hall P, et al. Long-term effectiveness of a staged assessment for paediatric problematic severe asthma. Eur Respir J. 2012;40(1):264–7.

82. Konradsen JR, Nordlund B, Lidegran M, Pedroletti C, Gronlund H, van Hage M, et al. Problematic severe asthma: a proposed approach to identifying children who are severely resistant to therapy. Pediatr Allergy Immunol. 2011;22(1 Pt 1):9–18.

83. Silkoff PE, Lent AM, Busacker AA, Katial RK, Balzar S, Strand M, et al. Exhaled nitric oxide identifies the persistent eosinophilic phenotype in severe refractory asthma. J Allergy Clin Immunol. 2005;116(6):1249–55.

84. Tseliou E, Bessa V, Hillas G, Delimpoura V, Papadaki G, Roussos C, et al. Exhaled nitric oxide and exhaled breath condensate pH in severe refractory asthma. Chest. 2010;138(1):107–13.

85. Michils A, Baldassarre S, Van Muylem A. Exhaled nitric oxide and asthma control: a longitudinal study in unselected patients. Eur Respir J. 2008;31(3):539–46.

86. Jones SL, Kittelson J, Cowan JO, Flannery EM, Hancox RJ, McLachlan CR, et al. The predictive value of exhaled nitric oxide measurements in assessing changes in asthma control. Am J Respir Crit Care Med. 2001;164(5):738–43.

87. Gelb AF, Flynn Taylor C, Shinar CM, Gutierrez C, Zamel N. Role of spirometry and exhaled nitric oxide to predict exacerbations in treated asthmatics. Chest. 2006;129(6):1492–9.

88. van der Valk RJ, Baraldi E, Stern G, Frey U, de Jongste JC. Daily exhaled nitric oxide measurements and asthma exacerbations in children. Allergy. 2012;67(2):265–71.

89. Brzozowska A, Majak P, Jerzynska J, Smejda K, Bobrowska-Korzeniowska M, Stelmach W, et al. Exhaled nitric oxide correlates with IL-2, MCP-1, PDGF-BB and TIMP-2 in exhaled breath condensate of children with refractory asthma. Postepy Dermatol Alergol. 2015;32(2):107–13.

90. Gomersal T, Harnan S, Essat M, Tappenden P, Wong R, Lawson R, et al. A systematic review of fractional exhaled nitric oxide in the routine management of childhood asthma. Pediatr Pulmonol. 2016;51(3):316–28.

91. Pike K, Selby A, Price S, Warner J, Connett G, Legg J, et al. Exhaled nitric oxide monitoring does not reduce exacerbation frequency or inhaled corticosteroid dose in paediatric asthma: a randomised controlled trial. Clin Respir J. 2013;7(2):204–13.

92. Peirsman EJ, Carvelli TJ, Hage PY, Hanssens LS, Pattyn L, Raes MM, et al. Exhaled nitric oxide in childhood allergic asthma management: a randomised controlled trial. Pediatr Pulmonol. 2014;49(7):624–31.

93. Petsky HL, Li AM, Au CT, Kynaston JA, Turner C, Chang AB. Management based on exhaled nitric oxide levels adjusted for atopy reduces asthma exacerbations in children: a dual centre randomized controlled trial. Pediatr Pulmonol. 2015;50(6):535–43.

94. Shaw DE, Berry MA, Hargadon B, McKenna S, Shelley MJ, Green RH, et al. Association between neutrophilic airway inflammation and airflow limitation in adults with asthma. Chest. 2007;132(6):1871–5.

95. Szefler SJ, Mitchell H, Sorkness CA, Gergen PJ, O'Connor GT, Morgan WJ, et al. Management of asthma based on exhaled nitric oxide in addition to guideline-based treatment for inner-city adolescents and young adults: a randomised controlled trial. Lancet. 2008;372(9643):1065–72.

96. Calhoun WJ, Ameredes BT, King TS, Icitovic N, Bleecker ER, Castro M, et al. Comparison of physician-, biomarker-, and symptom-based strategies for adjustment of inhaled corticosteroid therapy in adults with asthma: the BASALT randomized controlled trial. JAMA. 2012;308(10):987–97.

97. Petsky HL, Cates CJ, Lasserson TJ, Li AM, Turner C, Kynaston JA, et al. A systematic review and meta-analysis: tailoring asthma treatment on eosinophilic markers (exhaled nitric oxide or sputum eosinophils). Thorax. 2012;67(3):199–208.

98. Essat M, Harnan S, Gomersall T, Tappenden P, Wong R, Pavord I, et al. Fractional exhaled nitric oxide for the management of asthma in adults: a systematic review. Eur Respir J. 2016;47(3):751–68.

99. Malerba M, Ragnoli B, Radaeli A, Ricciardolo FLM. Long-term adjustment of stable asthma treatment with fractional exhaled nitric oxide and sputum eosinophils. Eur J Inflamm. 2012;10(3):383–92.

100. Gibson PG. Using fractional exhaled nitric oxide to guide asthma therapy: design and methodological issues for ASthma TReatment ALgorithm studies. Clin Exp Allergy. 2009;39(4):478–90.

101. Cowan DC, Taylor DR, Peterson LE, Cowan JO, Palmay R, Williamson A, et al. Biomarker-based asthma phenotypes of corticosteroid response. J Allergy Clin Immunol. 2015;135(4):877–83.e1.

102. Kharitonov SA, Yates DH, Barnes PJ. Inhaled glucocorticoids decrease nitric oxide in exhaled air of asthmatic patients. Am J Respir Crit Care Med. 1996;153(1):454–7.

103. Parulekar AD, Diamant Z, Hanania NA. Role of T2 inflammation biomarkers in severe asthma. Curr Opin Pulm Med. 2016;22(1):59–68.

104. Silkoff PE, Laviolette M, Singh D, FitzGerald JM, Kelsen S, Backer V, et al. Longitudinal stability of asthma characteristics and biomarkers from the Airways Disease Endotyping for Personalized Therapeutics (ADEPT) study. Respir Res. 2016; 17:43.

105. Kharitonov SA, Gonio F, Kelly C, Meah S, Barnes PJ. Reproducibility of exhaled nitric oxide measurements in healthy and asthmatic adults and children. Eur Respir J. 2003;21(3):433–8.

106. Ekroos H, Karjalainen J, Sarna S, Laitinen LA, Sovijarvi AR. Short-term variability of exhaled nitric oxide in young male patients with mild asthma and in healthy subjects. Respir Med. 2002;96(11):895–900.

107. Thijs W, de Mutsert R, le Cessie S, Hiemstra PS, Rosendaal FR, Middeldorp S, et al. Reproducibility of exhaled nitric oxide measurements in overweight and obese adults. BMC Res Notes. 2014;7:775.

108. Buchvald F, Eiberg H, Bisgaard H. Heterogeneity of FeNO response to inhaled steroid in asthmatic children. Clin Exp Allergy. 2003;33(12):1735–40.

109. Hanania NA, Wenzel S, Rosen K, Hsieh HJ, Mosesova S, Choy DF, et al. Exploring the effects of omalizumab in allergic asthma: an analysis of biomarkers in the EXTRA study. Am J Respir Crit Care Med. 2013;187(8):804–11.

110. Sorkness CA, Wildfire JJ, Calatroni A, Mitchell HE, Busse WW, O'Connor GT, et al. Reassessment of omalizumab-dosing strategies and pharmacodynamics in inner-city children and adolescents. J Allergy Clin Immunol Pract. 2013;1(2):163–71.

111. Wenzel S, Ford L, Pearlman D, Spector S, Sher L, Skobieranda F, et al. Dupilumab in persistent asthma with elevated eosinophil levels. N Engl J Med. 2013;368(26):2455–66.

112. Luo J, Liu D, Liu CT. The efficacy and safety of antiinterleukin 13, a monoclonal antibody, in adult patients with asthma: a systematic review and meta-analysis. Medicine. 2016;95(6):e2556.

113. American Thoracic S, European RS. ATS/ERS recommendations for standardized procedures for the online and offline measurement of exhaled lower respiratory nitric oxide and nasal nitric oxide, 2005. Am J Respir Crit Care Med. 2005;171(8):912–30.

114. Olin AC, Bake B, Toren K. Fraction of exhaled nitric oxide at 50 mL/s: reference values for adult lifelong never-smokers. Chest. 2007;131(6):1852–6.

115. Olin AC, Rosengren A, Thelle DS, Lissner L, Bake B, Toren K. Height, age, and atopy are associated with fraction of exhaled nitric oxide in a large adult general population sample. Chest. 2006;130(5):1319–25.

116. Grob NM, Dweik RA. Exhaled nitric oxide in asthma. From diagnosis, to monitoring, to screening: are we there yet? Chest. 2008;133(4):837–9.

117. Buchvald F, Baraldi E, Carraro S, Gaston B, De Jongste J, Pijnenburg MW, et al. Measurements of exhaled nitric oxide in healthy subjects age 4 to 17 years. J Allergy Clin Immunol. 2005;115(6):1130–6.

118. Olivieri M, Talamini G, Corradi M, Perbellini L, Mutti A, Tantucci C, et al. Reference values for exhaled nitric oxide (reveno) study. Respir Res. 2006;7:94.

119. Travers J, Marsh S, Aldington S, Williams M, Shirtcliffe P, Pritchard A, et al. Reference ranges for exhaled nitric oxide derived from a random community survey of adults. Am J Respir Crit Care Med. 2007;176(3):238–42.

120. Dressel H, de la Motte D, Reichert J, Ochmann U, Petru R, Angerer P, et al. Exhaled nitric oxide: independent effects of atopy, smoking, respiratory tract infection, gender and height. Respir Med. 2008;102(7):962–9.

121. Kovesi T, Kulka R, Dales R. Exhaled nitric oxide concentration is affected by age, height, and race in healthy 9- to 12-year-old children. Chest. 2008;133(1):169–75.

122. Wong GW, Liu EK, Leung TF, Yung E, Ko FW, Hui DS, et al. High levels and gender difference of exhaled nitric oxide in Chinese schoolchildren. Clin Exp Allergy. 2005;35(7):889–93.

123. Malmberg LP, Petays T, Haahtela T, Laatikainen T, Jousilahti P, Vartiainen E, et al. Exhaled nitric oxide in healthy nonatopic school-age children: determinants and height-adjusted reference values. Pediatr Pulmonol. 2006;41(7):635–42.

124. Jacinto T, Alving K, Correia R, Costa-Pereira A, Fonseca J. Setting reference values for exhaled nitric oxide: a systematic review. Clin Respir J. 2013;7(2):113–20.

125. Ludviksdottir D, Diamant Z, Alving K, Bjermer L, Malinovschi A. Clinical aspects of using exhaled NO in asthma diagnosis and management. Clin Respir J. 2012;6(4):193–207.

126. Saito J, Sato S, Fukuhara A, Sato Y, Nikaido T, Inokoshi Y, et al. Association of asthma education with asthma control evaluated by asthma control test, FEV1, and fractional exhaled nitric oxide. J Asthma. 2013;50(1):97–102.

127. Horvath I, Hunt J, Barnes PJ, Alving K, Antczak A, Baraldi E, et al. Exhaled breath condensate: methodological recommendations and unresolved questions. Eur Respir J. 2005;26(3):523–48.

128. Kietzmann D, Kahl R, Muller M, Burchardi H, Kettler D. Hydrogen peroxide in expired breath condensate of patients with acute respiratory failure and with ARDS. Intensive Care Med. 1993;19(2):78–81.

129. Effros RM, Hoagland KW, Bosbous M, Castillo D, Foss B, Dunning M, et al. Dilution of respiratory solutes in exhaled condensates. Am J Respir Crit Care Med. 2002;165(5):663–9.

130. Scheideler L, Manke HG, Schwulera U, Inacker O, Hammerle H. Detection of nonvolatile macromolecules in breath. A possible diagnostic tool? Am Rev Respir Dis. 1993;148(3):778–84.

131. Melo REPT, Solé D. <Exhaled breath temperature, a new biomarker in asthma control: a pilot study>. J Bras Pneumol. 2010;36(6):693–9.

132. Garcia G, Bergna M, Uribe E, Yanez A, Soriano JB. Increased exhaled breath temperature in subjects with uncontrolled asthma. Int J Tuberc Lung Dis. 2013;17(7):969–72.

133. Leonardi S, Cuppari C, Lanzafame A, Attardo D, Tardino L, Parisi G, et al. Exhaled breath temperature in asthmatic children. J Biol Regul Homeost Agents. 2015;29(2 Suppl 1):47–54.

134. Piacentini GL, Peroni D, Crestani E, Zardini F, Bodini A, Costella S, Boner AL. Exhaled air temperature in asthma: methods and relationship with markers of disease. Clin Exp Allergy. 2007;37(3):415–9.

135. Paredi P, Kharitonov SA, Barnes PJ. Correlation of exhaled breath temperature with bronchial blood flow in asthma. Respir Res. 2005;6:15.

136. Piacentini GLPD, Bodini A, Corradi M, Boner AL. Exhaled breath temperature as a marker of airway remodelling in asthma: a preliminary study. Allergy. 2008;63(4):484–5.

137. Crespo Lessmann A, Giner J, Torrego A, Mateus E, Torrejon M, Belda A, et al. Usefulness of the exhaled breath temperature plateau in asthma patients. Respiration. 2015;90(2):111–7.

138. Hamill L, Ferris K, Kapande K, McConaghy L, Douglas I, McGovern V, et al. Exhaled breath temperature measurement and asthma control in children prescribed inhaled corticosteroids: a cross sectional study. Pediatr Pulmonol. 2016;51(1):13–21.

139. Svensson H, Bjermer L, Tufvesson E. Exhaled breath temperature in asthmatics and controls after eucapnic voluntary hyperventilation and a methacholine challenge test. Respiration. 2014;87(2):149–57.

140. Vermeulen S, Barreto M, La Penna F, Prete A, Martella S, Biagiarelli F, et al. Exhaled breath temperature in children: reproducibility and influencing factors. J Asthma. 2014;51(7):743–50.

141. Barreto M, Piacentini G, Chiossi L, Ruggeri F, Caiazzo I, Campisano M, et al. Tidal-breathing measurement of exhaled breath temperature (EBT) in schoolchildren. Pediatr Pulmonol. 2014;49(12):1196–204.

142. Prince PBM, Boulet LP. A fast, simple, and inexpensive method to collect exhaled breath condensate for pH determination. Ann Allergy Asthma Immunol. 2006;97(5):622–7.

143. Paget-Brown AO, Ngamtrakulpanit L, Smith A, Bunyan D, Hom S, Nguyen A, et al. Normative data for pH of exhaled breath condensate. Chest. 2006;129(2):426–30.

144. Effros RM, Casaburi R, Porszasz J, Rehan V. Why conventional exhaled breath condensate pH studies cannot provide reliable estimates of airway acidification. Chest. 2011;140(4):1099.

145. Hunt JF, Fang K, Malik R, Snyder A, Malhotra N, Platts-Mills TA, Gaston B. Endogenous airway acidification. Implications for asthma pathophysiology. Am J Respir Crit Care Med. 2000;161(3 Pt 1):694–9.

146. Antus B, Barta I, Kullmann T, Lazar Z, Valyon M, Horvath I, et al. Assessment of exhaled breath condensate pH in exacerbations of asthma and chronic obstructive pulmonary disease: a longitudinal study. Am J Respir Crit Care Med. 2010;182(12):1492–7.

147. Fitzpatrick AM, Holbrook JT, Wei CY, Brown MS, Wise RA, Teague WG, et al. Exhaled breath condensate pH does not discriminate asymptomatic gastroesophageal reflux or the response to lansoprazole treatment in children with poorly controlled asthma. J Allergy Clin Immunol Pract. 2014;2(5):579–86.e7.

148. Bikov A, Galffy G, Tamasi L, Lazar Z, Losonczy G, Horvath I. Exhaled breath condensate pH is influenced by respiratory droplet dilution. J Breath Res. 2012;6(4):046002.

149. Liu L, Teague WG, Erzurum S, Fitzpatrick A, Mantri S, Dweik RA, et al. Determinants of exhaled breath condensate pH in a large population with asthma. Chest. 2011;139(2):328–36.

150. Leung TF, Li CY, Yung E, Liu EK, Lam CW, Wong GW. Clinical and technical factors affecting pH and other biomarkers in exhaled breath condensate. Pediatr Pulmonol. 2006;41(1):87–94.

151. von Jagwitz M, Pessler F, Akmatov M, Li J, Range U, Vogelberg C. Reduced breath condensate pH in asymptomatic children with prior wheezing as a risk factor for asthma. J Allergy Clin Immunol. 2011;128(1):50–5.

152. Caffarelli C, Dascola CP, Peroni D, Rico S, Stringari G, Varini M, et al. Airway acidification in childhood asthma exacerbations. Allergy Asthma Proc. 2014;35(3):51–6.

153. Tomasiak-Lozowska MM, Zietkowski Z, Przeslaw K, Tomasiak M, Skiepko R, Bodzenta-Lukaszyk A. Inflammatory markers and acid-base equilibrium in exhaled breath condensate of stable and unstable asthma patients. Int Arch Allergy Immunol. 2012;159(2):121–9.

154. Kane B, Borrill Z, Southworth T, Woodcock A, Singh D. Reduced exhaled breath condensate pH in asthmatic smokers using inhaled corticosteroids. Respirology. 2009;14(3):419–23.

155. Davies KJ. Oxidative stress: the paradox of aerobic life. Biochem Soc Symp. 1995;61:1–31.

156. Conner EM, Grisham MB. Inflammation, free radicals, and antioxidants. Nutrition. 1996;12(4):274–7.

157. Jöbsis Q, Raatgeep HC, Hermans PW, de Jongste JC. Hydrogen peroxide in exhaled air is increased in stable asthmatic children. Eur Respir J. 1997;10(3):519–21.

158. Antczak A, Nowak D, Shariati B, Król M, Piasecka G, Kurmanowska Z. Increased hydrogen peroxide and thiobarbituric acid-reactive products in expired breath condensate of asthmatic patients. Eur Respir J. 1997;10(6):1235–41.

159. Emelyanov A, Fedoseev G, Abulimity A, Rudinski K, Fedoulov A, Karabanov A, et al. Elevated concentrations of exhaled hydrogen peroxide in asthmatic patients. Chest. 2001;120(4):1136–9.

160. Loukides S, Bouros D, Papatheodorou G, Panagou P, Siafakas NM. The relationships among hydrogen peroxide in expired breath condensate, airway inflammation, and asthma severity. Chest. 2002;121(2):338–46.

161. Al-Obaidy AH, Al-Samarai AG. Exhaled breath condensate pH and hydrogen peroxide as non-invasive markers for asthma. Saudi Med J. 2007;28(12):1860–3.

162. Caffarelli C, Calcinai E, Rinaldi L, Povesi Dascola C, Terracciano L, Corradi M. Hydrogen peroxide in exhaled breath condensate in asthmatic children during acute exacerbation and after treatment. Respiration. 2012;84(4):291–8.

163. Murata K, Fujimoto K, Kitaguchi Y, Horiuchi T, Kubo K, Honda T. Hydrogen peroxide content and pH of expired breath condensate from patients with asthma and COPD. COPD. 2014;11(1):81–7.

164. Warwick G, Thomas PS, Yates DH. Non-invasive biomarkers in exacerbations of obstructive lung disease. Respirology. 2013;18(5):874–84.

165. Trischler J, Merkel N, Konitzer S, Muller CM, Unverzagt S, Lex C. Fractionated breath condensate sampling: H(2)O(2) concentrations of the alveolar fraction may be related to asthma control in children. Respir Res. 2012;13:14.

166. Al Obaidi AH, Al Samarai AM. Biochemical markers as a response guide for steroid therapy in asthma. J Asthma. 2008;45(5):425–8.

167. Teng Y, Sun P, Zhang J, Yu R, Bai J, Yao X, et al. Hydrogen peroxide in exhaled breath condensate in patients with asthma: a promising biomarker? Chest. 2011;140(1):108–16.

168. Robroeks CM, van Vliet D, Jobsis Q, Braekers R, Rijkers GT, Wodzig WK, et al. Prediction of asthma exacerbations in children: results of a one-year prospective study. Clin Exp Allergy. 2012;42(5):792–8.

169. Sood A, Qualls C, Seagrave J, McDonald J, Shohreh R, Chiavaroli A, et al. Effect of allergen inhalation on airway oxidant stress, using exhaled breath condensate 8-isoprostane, in mild asthma. J Asthma. 2013;50(5):449–56.

170. Koskela HO, Purokivi MK, Nieminen RM, Moilanen E. Asthmatic cough and airway oxidative stress. Respir Physiol Neurobiol. 2012;181(3):346–50.

171. Montuschi P, Corradi M, Ciabattoni G, Nightingale J, Kharitonov SA, Barnes PJ. Increased 8-isoprostane, a marker of oxidative stress, in exhaled condensate of asthma patients. Am J Respir Crit Care Med. 1999;160(1):216–20.

172. Baraldi E, Ghiro L, Piovan V, Carraro S, Ciabattoni G, Barnes PJ, et al. Increased exhaled 8-isoprostane in childhood asthma. Chest. 2003;124(1):25–31.

173. Mondino C, Ciabattoni G, Koch P, Pistelli R, Trove A, Barnes PJ, et al. Effects of inhaled corticosteroids on exhaled leukotrienes and prostanoids in asthmatic children. J Allergy Clin Immunol. 2004;114(4):761–7.

174. Zanconato S, Carraro S, Corradi M, Alinovi R, Pasquale MF, Piacentini G, et al. Leukotrienes and 8-isoprostane in exhaled breath condensate of children with stable and unstable asthma. J Allergy Clin Immunol. 2004;113(2):257–63.

175. Shahid SK, Kharitonov SA, Wilson NM, Bush A, Barnes PJ. Exhaled 8-isoprostane in childhood asthma. Respir Res. 2005;6:79.

176. Samitas K, Chorianopoulos D, Vittorakis S, Zervas E, Economidou E, Papatheodorou G, et al. Exhaled

cysteinyl-leukotrienes and 8-isoprostane in patients with asthma and their relation to clinical severity. Respir Med. 2009;103(5):750–6.

177. Caballero Balanzá S, Martorell Aragonés A, Cerdá Mir JC, Belda Ramírez J, Navarro Iváñez R, Navarro Soriano A, et al. Leukotriene B4 and 8-isoprostane in exhaled breath condensate of children with episodic and persistent asthma. J Investig Allergol Clin Immunol. 2010;20(3):237–43.

178. Hasan RA, O'Brien E, Mancuso P. Lipoxin A(4) and 8-isoprostane in the exhaled breath condensate of children hospitalized for status asthmaticus. Pediatr Crit Med. 2012;13(2):141–5.

179. Carraro S, Cogo PE, Isak I, Simonato M, Corradi M, Carnielli VP, et al. EIA and GC/MS analysis of 8-isoprostane in EBC of children with problematic asthma. Eur Respir J. 2010;35(6):1364–9.

180. Keskin O, Balaban S, Keskin M, Kucukosmanoglu E, Gogebakan B, Ozkars MY, et al. Relationship between exhaled leukotriene and 8-isoprostane levels and asthma severity, asthma control level, and asthma control test score. Allergol Immunopathol. 2014;42(3):191–7.

181. Brussino L, Badiu I, Sciascia S, Bugiani M, Heffler E, Guida G, et al. Oxidative stress and airway inflammation after allergen challenge evaluated by exhaled breath condensate analysis. Clin Exp Allergy. 2010;40(11):1642–7.

182. Piotrowski WJ, Majewski S, Marczak J, Kurmanowska Z, Gorski P, Antczak A. Exhaled breath 8-isoprostane as a marker of asthma severity. Arch Med Sci. 2012;8(3):515–20.

183. Keskin O, Uluca U, Keskin M, Gogebakan B, Kucukosmanoglu E, Ozkars MY, et al. The efficacy of single-high dose inhaled corticosteroid versus oral prednisone treatment on exhaled leukotriene and 8-isoprostane levels in mild to moderate asthmatic children with asthma exacerbation. Allergol Immunopathol. 2016;44(2):138–48.

184. Liu J, Thomas PS. Exhaled breath condensate as a method of sampling airway nitric oxide and other markers of inflammation. Med Sci Monit. 2005;11(8):MT53–62.

185. Ganas K, Loukides S, Papatheodorou G, Panagou P, Kalogeropoulos N. Total nitrite/nitrate in expired breath condensate of patients with asthma. Respir Med. 2001;95(8):649–54.

186. Corradi M, Pesci A, Casana R, Alinovi R, Goldoni M, Vettori MV, et al. Nitrate in exhaled breath condensate of patients with different airway diseases. Nitric Oxide. 2003;8(1):26–30.

187. Ratnawati, Morton J, Henry RL, Thomas PS. Exhaled breath condensate nitrite/nitrate and pH in relation to pediatric asthma control and exhaled nitric oxide. Pediatr Pulmonol. 2006;41(10):929–36.

188. Zetterquist W, Marteus H, Hedlin G, Alving K. Increased exhaled nitrite in children with allergic asthma is not related to nitric oxide formation. Clin Respir J. 2008;2(3):166–74.

189. Bouzigon E, Monier F, Boussaha M, Le Moual N, Huyvaert H, Matran R, et al. Associations between nitric oxide synthase genes and exhaled NO-related phenotypes according to asthma status. PLoS One. 2012;7(5):e36672.

190. Hauswirth DW, Sundy JS, Mervin-Blake S, Fernandez CA, Patch KB, Alexander KM, et al. Normative values for exhaled breath condensate pH and its relationship to exhaled nitric oxide in healthy African Americans. J Allergy Clin Immunol. 2008;122(1):101–6.

191. Rihak V, Zatloukal P, Chladkova J, Zimulova A, Havlinova Z, Chladek J. Nitrite in exhaled breath condensate as a marker of nitrossative stress in the airways of patients with asthma, COPD, and idiopathic pulmonary fibrosis. J Clin Lab Anal. 2010;24(5):317–22.

192. Malinovschi A, Pizzimenti S, Sciascia S, Heffler E, Badiu I, Rolla G. Exhaled breath condensate nitrates, but not nitrites or FENO, relate to asthma control. Respir Med. 2011;105(7):1007–13.

193. Scott JA, North ML, Rafii M, Huang H, Pencharz P, Subbarao P, et al. Asymmetric dimethylarginine is increased in asthma. Am J Respir Crit Care Med. 2011;184(7):779–85.

194. Carraro S, Giordano G, Piacentini G, Kantar A, Moser S, Cesca L, et al. Asymmetric dimethylarginine in exhaled breath condensate and serum of children with asthma. Chest. 2013;144(2):405–10.

195. Samuelsson B, Granstrom E, Green K, Hamberg M, Hammarstrom S. Prostaglandins. Annu Rev Biochem. 1975;44:669–95.

196. Montuschi P, Barnes PJ. Analysis of exhaled breath condensate for monitoring airway inflammation. Trends Pharmacol Sci. 2002;23(5):232–7.

197. Montuschi P, Barnes PJ. Exhaled leukotrienes and prostaglandins in asthma. J Allergy Clin Immunol. 2002;109(4):615–20.

198. Samuelsson B. Leukotrienes: mediators of immediate hypersensitivity reactions and inflammation. Science. 1983;220(4597):568–75.

199. Montuschi P, Sala A, Dahlen S-E, Folco G. Pharmacological modulation of the leukotriene pathway in allergic airway disease. Drug Discov Today. 2007;12;404.

200. Wardlaw AJ, Hay H, Cromwell O, Collins JV, Kay AB. Leukotrienes, LTC4 and LTB4, in bronchoalveolar lavage in bronchial asthma and other respiratory diseases. J Allergy Clin Immunol. 1989;84(1):19–26.

201. Claesson HE, Odlander B, Jakobsson PJ. Leukotriene B4 in the immune system. Int J Immunopharmacol. 1992;14(3):441–9.

202. Hallstrand TS, Henderson WR Jr. An update on the role of leukotrienes in asthma. Curr Opin Allergy Clin Immunol. 2010;10(1):60–6.

203. Holgate ST, Peters-Golden M, Panettieri RA, Henderson WR Jr. Roles of cysteinyl leukotrienes in airway inflammation, smooth muscle function, and remodeling. J Allergy Clin Immunol. 2003;111(1 Suppl):S18–34. discussion S-6

204. Ono E, Mita H, Taniguchi M, Higashi N, Tsuburai T, Hasegawa M, et al. Increase in inflammatory mediator concentrations in exhaled breath condensate

after allergen inhalation. J Allergy Clin Immunol. 2008;122(4):768–73.e1.

205. Antczak A, Montuschi P, Kharitonov S, Gorski P, Barnes PJ. Increased exhaled cysteinyl-leukotrienes and 8-isoprostane in aspirin-induced asthma. Am J Respir Crit Care Med. 2002;166(3):301–6.

206. Montuschi P, Mondino C, Koch P, Barnes PJ, Ciabattoni G. Effects of a leukotriene receptor antagonist on exhaled leukotriene E4 and prostanoids in children with asthma. J Allergy Clin Immunol. 2006;118(2):347–53.

207. Kielbasa B, Moeller A, Sanak M, Hamacher J, Hutterli M, Cmiel A, et al. Eicosanoids in exhaled breath condensates in the assessment of childhood asthma. Pediatr Allergy Immunol. 2008;19(7):660–9.

208. Hanazawa T, Kharitonov SA, Barnes PJ. Increased nitrotyrosine in exhaled breath condensate of patients with asthma. Am J Respir Crit Care Med. 2000;162(4 Pt 1):1273–6.

209. Cap P, Chladek J, Pehal F, Maly M, Petru V, Barnes PJ, et al. Gas chromatography/mass spectrometry analysis of exhaled leukotrienes in asthmatic patients. Thorax. 2004;59(6):465–70.

210. Baraldi E, Carraro S, Alinovi R, Pesci A, Ghiro L, Bodini A, et al. Cysteinyl leukotrienes and 8-isoprostane in exhaled breath condensate of children with asthma exacerbations. Thorax. 2003;58(6):505–9.

211. Laberge S, El Bassam S. Cytokines, structural cells of the lungs and airway inflammation. Paediatr Respir Rev. 2004;5(Suppl A):S41–5.

212. Shahid SK, Kharitonov SA, Wilson NM, Bush A, Barnes PJ. Increased interleukin-4 and decreased interferon-gamma in exhaled breath condensate of children with asthma. Am J Respir Crit Care Med. 2002;165(9):1290–3.

213. Carpagnano GE, Resta O, Ventura MT, Amoruso AC, Di Gioia G, Giliberti T, et al. Airway inflammation in subjects with gastro-oesophageal reflux and gastro-oesophageal reflux-related asthma. J Intern Med. 2006;259(3):323–31.

214. Robroeks CM, van de Kant KD, Jobsis Q, Hendriks HJ, van Gent R, Wouters EF, et al. Exhaled nitric oxide and biomarkers in exhaled breath condensate indicate the presence, severity and control of childhood asthma. Clin Exp Allergy. 2007;37(9):1303–11.

215. Profita M, La Grutta S, Carpagnano E, Riccobono L, Di Giorgi R, Bonanno A, et al. Noninvasive methods for the detection of upper and lower airway inflammation in atopic children. J Allergy Clin Immunol. 2006;118(5):1068–74.

216. Carpagnano GE, Foschino Barbaro MP, Cagnazzo M, Di Gioia G, Giliberti T, Di Matteo C, et al. Use of exhaled breath condensate in the study of airway inflammation after hypertonic saline solution challenge. Chest. 2005;128(5):3159–66.

217. Matsunaga K, Yanagisawa S, Ichikawa T, Ueshima K, Akamatsu K, Hirano T, et al. Airway cytokine expression measured by means of protein array in exhaled breath condensate: correlation with physio-

logic properties in asthmatic patients. J Allergy Clin Immunol. 2006;118(1):84–90.

218. Ojoo JC, Mulrennan SA, Kastelik JA, Morice AH, Redington AE. Exhaled breath condensate pH and exhaled nitric oxide in allergic asthma and in cystic fibrosis. Thorax. 2005;60(1):22–6.

219. Gluck J, Rymarczyk B, Kasprzak M, Rogala B. Increased levels of interleukin-33 and thymic stromal lymphopoietin in exhaled breath condensate in chronic bronchial asthma. Int Arch Allergy Immunol. 2016;169(1):51–6.

220. Zietkowski Z, Skiepko R, Tomasiak MM, Bodzenta-Lukaszyk A. Endothelin-1 in exhaled breath condensate of stable and unstable asthma patients. Respir Med. 2008;102(3):470–4.

221. Zietkowski Z, Tomasiak MM, Skiepko R, Bodzenta-Lukaszyk A. RANTES in exhaled breath condensate of stable and unstable asthma patients. Respir Med. 2008;102(8):1198–202.

222. Zietkowski Z, Tomasiak-Lozowska MM, Skiepko R, Zietkowska E, Bodzenta-Lukaszyk A. Eotaxin-1 in exhaled breath condensate of stable and unstable asthma patients. Respir Res. 2010;11:110.

223. Wu D, Zhou J, Bi H, Li L, Gao W, Huang M, et al. CCL11 as a potential diagnostic marker for asthma? J Asthma. 2014;51(8):847–54.

224. Huszar E, Vass G, Vizi E, Csoma Z, Barat E, Molnar Vilagos G, et al. Adenosine in exhaled breath condensate in healthy volunteers and in patients with asthma. Eur Respir J. 2002;20(6):1393–8.

225. Greenwald R, Fitzpatrick AM, Gaston B, Marozkina NV, Erzurum S, Teague WG. Breath formate is a marker of airway S-nitrosothiol depletion in severe asthma. PLoS One. 2010;5(7):e11919.

226. Simpson JL, Scott RJ, Boyle MJ, Gibson PG. Differential proteolytic enzyme activity in eosinophilic and neutrophilic asthma. Am J Respir Crit Care Med. 2005;172(5):559–65.

227. Corradi M, Folesani G, Andreoli R, Manini P, Bodini A, Piacentini G, et al. Aldehydes and glutathione in exhaled breath condensate of children with asthma exacerbation. Am J Respir Crit Care Med. 2003;167(3):395–9.

228. Zietkowski Z, Tomasiak-Lozowska MM, Skiepko R, Mroczko B, Szmitkowski M, Bodzenta-Lukaszyk A. High-sensitivity C-reactive protein in the exhaled breath condensate and serum in stable and unstable asthma. Respir Med. 2009;103(3):379–85.

229. Grob NM, Aytckin M, Dweik RA. Biomarkers in exhaled breath condensate: a review of collection, processing and analysis. J Breath Res. 2008;2(3):037004.

230. Bloemen K, Van Den Heuvel R, Govarts E, Hooyberghs J, Nelen V, Witters E, et al. A new approach to study exhaled proteins as potential biomarkers for asthma. Clin Exp Allergy. 2011;41(3):346–56.

231. Bartoli ML, Novelli F, Costa F, Malagrino L, Melosini L, Bacci E, et al. Malondialdehyde in exhaled breath condensate as a marker of oxida-

tive stress in different pulmonary diseases. Mediat Inflamm. 2011;2011:891752.

232. Motta A, Paris D, D'Amato M, Melck D, Calabrese C, Vitale C, et al. NMR metabolomic analysis of exhaled breath condensate of asthmatic patients at two different temperatures. J Proteome Res. 2014;13(12):6107–20.

233. Klaassen EM, van de Kant KD, Jobsis Q, Penders J, van Schooten FJ, Quaak M, et al. Integrative genomic analysis identifies a role for intercellular adhesion molecule 1 in childhood asthma. Pediatr Allergy Immunol. 2014;25(2):166–72.

234. Miekisch W, Schubert JK, Noeldge-Schomburg GF. Diagnostic potential of breath analysis—focus on volatile organic compounds. Clin Chim Acta. 2004;347(1–2):25–39.

235. Buszewski B, Kesy M, Ligor T, Amann A. Human exhaled air analytics: biomarkers of diseases. Biomedical Chromatogr. 2007;21(6):553–66.

236. van de Kant KD, van der Sande LJ, Jobsis Q, van Schayck OC, Dompeling E. Clinical use of exhaled volatile organic compounds in pulmonary diseases: a systematic review. Respir Res. 2012;13:117.

237. Olopade CO, Zakkar M, Swedler WI, Rubinstein I. Exhaled pentane levels in acute asthma. Chest. 1997;111(4):862–5.

238. Caldeira M, Perestrelo R, Barros AS, Bilelo MJ, Morete A, Camara JS, et al. Allergic asthma exhaled breath metabolome: a challenge for comprehensive two-dimensional gas chromatography. J Chromatogr A. 2012;1254:87–97.

239. Smolinska A, Klaassen EM, Dallinga JW, van de Kant KD, Jobsis Q, Moonen EJ, et al. Profiling of volatile organic compounds in exhaled breath as a strategy to find early predictive signatures of asthma in children. PLoS One. 2014;9(4):e95668.

240. Dragonieri S, Schot R, Mertens BJ, Le Cessie S, Gauw SA, Spanevello A, et al. An electronic nose in the discrimination of patients with asthma and controls. J Allergy Clin Immunol. 2007;120(4):856–62.

241. Paredi P, Kharitonov SA, Barnes PJ. Elevation of exhaled ethane concentration in asthma. Am J Respir Crit Care Med. 2000;162(4 Pt 1):1450–4.

242. Fens N, Zwinderman AH, van der Schee MP, de Nijs SB, Dijkers E, Roldaan AC, et al. Exhaled breath profiling enables discrimination of chronic obstructive pulmonary disease and asthma. Am J Respir Crit Care Med. 2009;180(11):1076–82.

243. Timms C, Thomas PS, Yates DH. Detection of gastro-oesophageal reflux disease (GORD) in patients with obstructive lung disease using exhaled breath profiling. J Breath Res. 2012;6(1):016003.

244. Delfino RJ, Gong H, Linn WS, Hu Y, Pellizzari ED. Respiratory symptoms and peak expiratory flow in children with asthma in relation to volatile organic compounds in exhaled breath and ambient air. J Expo Anal Environ Epidemiol. 2003;13(5):348–63.

245. Robroeks CM, van Berkel JJ, Jobsis Q, van Schooten FJ, Dallinga JW, Wouters EF, et al. Exhaled volatile organic compounds predict exacerbations of child-

hood asthma in a 1-year prospective study. Eur Respir J. 2013;42(1):98–106.

246. van der Schee MP, Palmay R, Cowan JO, Taylor DR. Predicting steroid responsiveness in patients with asthma using exhaled breath profiling. Clin Exp Allergy. 2013;43(11):1217–25.

247. Sly PD, Boner AL, Bjorksten B, Bush A, Custovic A, Eigenmann PA, et al. Early identification of atopy in the prediction of persistent asthma in children. Lancet. 2008;372(9643):1100–6.

248. Simpson A, Tan VY, Winn J, Svensen M, Bishop CM, Heckerman DE, et al. Beyond atopy: multiple patterns of sensitization in relation to asthma in a birth cohort study. Am J Respir Crit Care Med. 2010;181(11):1200–6.

249. Stoltz DJ, Jackson DJ, Evans MD, Gangnon RE, Tisler CJ, Gern JE, et al. Specific patterns of allergic sensitization in early childhood and asthma & rhinitis risk. Clin Exp Allergy. 2013;43(2):233–41.

250. Bousquet J, Wenzel S, Holgate S, Lumry W, Freeman P, Fox H. Predicting response to omalizumab, an anti-IgE antibody, in patients with allergic asthma. Chest. 2004;125(4):1378–86.

251. Wahn U, Martin C, Freeman P, Blogg M, Jimenez P. Relationship between pretreatment specific IgE and the response to omalizumab therapy. Allergy. 2009;64(12):1780–7.

252. Szefler SJ, Wenzel S, Brown R, Erzurum SC, Fahy JV, Hamilton RG, et al. Asthma outcomes: biomarkers. J Allergy Clin Immunol. 2012;129(3 Suppl):S9–23.

253. Peters MC, Mekonnen ZK, Yuan S, Bhakta NR, Woodruff PG, Fahy JV. Measures of gene expression in sputum cells can identify TH2-high and TH2-low subtypes of asthma. J Allergy Clin Immunol. 2014;133(2):388–94.

254. Tran TN, Khatry DB, Ke X, Ward CK, Gossage D. High blood eosinophil count is associated with more frequent asthma attacks in asthma patients. Ann Allergy Asthma Immunol. 2014;113(1):19–24.

255. Ulrik CS, Frederiksen J. Mortality and markers of risk of asthma death among 1,075 outpatients with asthma. Chest. 1995;108(1):10–5.

256. Malinovschi A, Fonseca JA, Jacinto T, Alving K, Janson C. Exhaled nitric oxide levels and blood eosinophil counts independently associate with wheeze and asthma events in National Health and Nutrition Examination Survey subjects. J Allergy Clin Immunol. 2013;132(4):821–7 e1-5.

257. Ulrik CS. Peripheral eosinophil counts as a marker of disease activity in intrinsic and extrinsic asthma. Clin Exp Allergy. 1995;25(9):820–7.

258. Taylor KJ, Luksza AR. Peripheral blood eosinophil counts and bronchial responsiveness. Thorax. 1987;42(6):452–6.

259. Szefler SJ, Phillips BR, Martinez FD, Chinchilli VM, Lemanske RF, Strunk RC, et al. Characterization of within-subject responses to fluticasone and montelukast in childhood asthma. J Allergy Clin Immunol. 2005;115(2):233–42.

260. Kupczyk M, Haque S, Middelveld RJ, Dahlen B, Dahlen SE, Investigators B. Phenotypic predictors of response to oral glucocorticosteroids in severe asthma. Respir Med. 2013;107(10):1521–30.

261. Castro M, Wenzel SE, Bleecker ER, Pizzichini E, Kuna P, Busse WW, et al. Benralizumab, an anti-interleukin 5 receptor alpha monoclonal antibody, versus placebo for uncontrolled eosinophilic asthma: a phase 2b randomised dose-ranging study. Lancet Respir Med. 2014;2(11):879–90.

262. Ortega HG, Liu MC, Pavord ID, Brusselle GG, FitzGerald JM, Chetta A, et al. Mepolizumab treatment in patients with severe eosinophilic asthma. N Engl J Med. 2014;371(13):1198–207.

263. Pavord ID, Korn S, Howarth P, Bleecker ER, Buhl R, Keene ON, et al. Mepolizumab for severe eosinophilic asthma (DREAM): a multicentre, double-blind, placebo-controlled trial. Lancet. 2012;380(9842):651–9.

264. Bel EH, Wenzel SE, Thompson PJ, Prazma CM, Keene ON, Yancey SW, et al. Oral glucocorticoid-sparing effect of mepolizumab in eosinophilic asthma. N Engl J Med. 2014;371(13):1189–97.

265. Nair P, Pizzichini MM, Kjarsgaard M, Inman MD, Efthimiadis A, Pizzichini E, et al. Mepolizumab for prednisone-dependent asthma with sputum eosinophilia. N Engl J Med. 2009;360(10):985–93.

266. Castro M, Mathur S, Hargreave F, Boulet LP, Xie F, Young J, et al. Reslizumab for poorly controlled, eosinophilic asthma: a randomized, placebo-controlled study. Am J Respir Crit Care Med. 2011;184(10):1125–32.

267. Busse W, Spector S, Rosén K, Wang Y, Alpan O. High eosinophil count: a potential biomarker for assessing successful omalizumab treatment effects. J Allergy Clin Immunol. 2013;132(2):485–6.e11.

268. Haldar P, Brightling CE, Hargadon B, Gupta S, Monteiro W, Sousa A, et al. Mepolizumab and exacerbations of refractory eosinophilic asthma. N Engl J Med. 2009;360(10):973–84.

269. Leckie MJ, ten Brinke A, Khan J, Diamant Z, O'Connor BJ, Walls CM, et al. Effects of an interleukin-5 blocking monoclonal antibody on eosinophils, airway hyper-responsiveness, and the late asthmatic response. Lancet. 2000;356(9248):2144–8.

270. Gauthier M, Ray A, Wenzel SE. Evolving concepts of asthma. Am J Respir Crit Care Med. 2015;192(6):660–8.

271. Takayama G, Arima K, Kanaji T, Toda S, Tanaka H, Shoji S, et al. Periostin: a novel component of subepithelial fibrosis of bronchial asthma downstream of IL-4 and IL-13 signals. J Allergy Clin Immunol. 2006;118(1):98–104.

272. Sidhu SS, Yuan S, Innes AL, Kerr S, Woodruff PG, Hou L, et al. Roles of epithelial cell-derived periostin in TGF-beta activation, collagen production, and collagen gel elasticity in asthma. Proc Natl Acad Sci U S A. 2010;107(32):14170–5.

273. Woodruff PG, Boushey HA, Dolganov GM, Barker CS, Yang YH, Donnelly S, et al. Genome-wide profiling identifies epithelial cell genes associated with asthma and with treatment response to corticosteroids. Proc Natl Acad Sci U S A. 2007;104(40):15858–63.

274. Yuyama N, Davies DE, Akaiwa M, Matsui K, Hamasaki Y, Suminami Y, et al. Analysis of novel disease-related genes in bronchial asthma. Cytokine. 2002;19(6):287–96.

275. Lopez-Guisa JM, Powers C, File D, Cochrane E, Jimenez N, Debley JS. Airway epithelial cells from asthmatic children differentially express proremodeling factors. J Allergy Clin Immunol. 2012;129(4):990–7. e6

276. Blanchard C, Mingler MK, McBride M, Putnam PE, Collins MH, Chang G, et al. Periostin facilitates eosinophil tissue infiltration in allergic lung and esophageal responses. Mucosal Immunol. 2008;1(4):289–96.

277. Conway SJ, Izuhara K, Kudo Y, Litvin J, Markwald R, Ouyang G, et al. The role of periostin in tissue remodeling across health and disease. Cell Mol Life Sci. 2014;71(7):1279–88.

278. Jia G, Erickson RW, Choy DF, Mosesova S, Wu LC, Solberg OD, et al. Periostin is a systemic biomarker of eosinophilic airway inflammation in asthmatic patients. J Allergy Clin Immunol. 2012;130(3):647–54. e10

279. Kanemitsu Y, Matsumoto H, Izuhara K, Tohda Y, Kita H, Horiguchi T, et al. Increased periostin associates with greater airflow limitation in patients receiving inhaled corticosteroids. J Allergy Clin Immunol. 2013;132(2):305–12. e3

280. Hanania NA, Noonan M, Corren J, Korenblat P, Zheng Y, Fischer SK, et al. Lebrikizumab in moderate-to-severe asthma: pooled data from two randomised placebo-controlled studies. Thorax. 2015;70(8):748–56.

281. Corren J, Lemanske RF, Hanania NA, Korenblat PE, Parsey MV, Arron JR, et al. Lebrikizumab treatment in adults with asthma. N Engl J Med. 2011;365(12):1088–98.

282. Masuoka M, Shiraishi H, Ohta S, Suzuki S, Arima K, Aoki S, et al. Periostin promotes chronic allergic inflammation in response to Th2 cytokines. J Clin Invest. 2012;122(7):2590–600.

283. Matsumoto H. Serum periostin: a novel biomarker for asthma management. Allergol Int. 2014;63(2):153–60.

284. Izuhara K, Matsumoto H, Ohta S, Ono J, Arima K, Ogawa M. Recent developments regarding periostin in bronchial asthma. Allergol Int. 2015;64(Suppl):S3–10.

285. Bobolea I, Barranco P, Del Pozo V, Romero D, Sanz V, Lopez-Carrasco V, et al. Sputum periostin in patients with different severe asthma phenotypes. Allergy. 2015;70(5):540–6.

286. Gorska K, Maskey-Warzechowska M, Nejman-Gryz P, Korczynski P, Prochorec-Sobieszek M, Krenke R. Comparative study of periostin expression in different respiratory samples in patients with asthma

and chronic obstructive pulmonary disease. Pol Arch Med Wewn. 2016;126(3):124–37.

287. Patil SP, Wisnivesky JP, Busse PJ, Halm EA, Li XM. Detection of immunological biomarkers correlated with asthma control and quality of life measurements in sera from chronic asthmatic patients. Ann Allergy Asthma Immunol. 2011;106(3):205–13.

288. Saad-El-Din Bessa S, Abo El-Magd GH, Mabrouk MM. Serum chemokines RANTES and monocyte chemoattractant protein-1 in Egyptian patients with atopic asthma: relationship to disease severity. Arch Med Res. 2012;43(1):36–41.

289. Chambers ES, Nanzer AM, Pfeffer PE, Richards DF, Timms PM, Martineau AR, et al. Distinct endotypes of steroid-resistant asthma characterized by IL-17A(high) and IFN-gamma(high) immunophenotypes: potential benefits of calcitriol. J Allergy Clin Immunol. 2015;136(3):628–37. e4

290. Ciprandi G, Cuppari C, Salpietro AM, Tosca MA, Rigoli L, Grasso L, et al. Serum IL-23 strongly and inversely correlates with FEV1 in asthmatic children. Int Arch Allergy Immunol. 2012;159(2):183–6.

291. Sziksz E, Kozma GT, Pallinger E, Komlosi ZI, Adori C, Kovacs L, et al. Galectin-9 in allergic airway inflammation and hyper-responsiveness in mice. Int Arch Allergy Immunol. 2010;151(4):308–17.

292. Niki T, Tsutsui S, Hirose S, Aradono S, Sugimoto Y, Takeshita K, et al. Galectin-9 is a high affinity IgE-binding lectin with anti-allergic effect by blocking IgE-antigen complex formation. J Biol Chem. 2009;284(47):32344–52.

293. Katoh S, Shimizu H, Obase Y, Oomizu S, Niki T, Ikeda M, et al. Preventive effect of galectin-9 on double-stranded RNA-induced airway hyperresponsiveness in an exacerbation model of mite antigen-induced asthma in mice. Exp Lung Res. 2013;39(10):453–62.

294. Hsu DK, Zuberi RI, Liu FT. Biochemical and biophysical characterization of human recombinant IgE-binding protein, an S-type animal lectin. J Biol Chem. 1992;267(20):14167–74.

295. Di Lella S, Sundblad V, Cerliani JP, Guardia CM, Estrin DA, Vasta GR, et al. When galectins recognize glycans: from biochemistry to physiology and back again. Biochemistry. 2011;50(37):7842–57.

296. Newlaczyl AU, Yu LG. Galectin-3—a jack-of-all-trades in cancer. Cancer Lett. 2011;313(2):123–8.

297. Mauri P, Riccio AM, Rossi R, Di Silvestre D, Benazzi L, De Ferrari L, et al. Proteomics of bronchial biopsies: galectin-3 as a predictive biomarker of airway remodelling modulation in omalizumab-treated severe asthma patients. Immunol Lett. 2014;162(1 Pt A):2–10.

298. Mosca T, Menezes MC, Dionigi PC, Stirbulov R, Forte WC. C3 and C4 complement system components as biomarkers in the intermittent atopic asthma diagnosis. J Pediatr. 2011;87(6):512–6.

299. Tang H, Fang Z, Sun Y, Li B, Shi Z, Chen J, et al. YKL-40 in asthmatic patients, and its correlations

with exacerbation, eosinophils and immunoglobulin E. Eur Respir J. 2010;35(4):757–60.

300. Specjalski K, Jassem E. YKL-40 protein is a marker of asthma. J Asthma. 2011;48(8):767–72.

301. Ezzat MH, Imam SS, Shaheen KY, Elbrhami EM. Serum OX40 ligand levels in asthmatic children: a potential biomarker of severity and persistence. Allergy Asthma Proc. 2011;32(4):313–8.

302. Tanju A, Cekmez F, Aydinoz S, Karademir F, Suleymanoglu S, Gocmen I. Association between clinical severity of childhood asthma and serum leptin levels. Indian J Pediatr. 2011;78(3):291–5.

303. Nishioka T, Uchida K, Meno K, Ishii T, Aoki T, Imada Y, et al. Alpha-1-antitrypsin and complement component C7 are involved in asthma exacerbation. Proteomics Clin Appl. 2008;2(1):46–54.

304. Rhim T, Choi YS, Nam BY, Uh ST, Park JS, Kim YH, et al. Plasma protein profiles in early asthmatic responses to inhalation allergen challenge. Allergy. 2009;64(1):47–54.

305. Singh A, Cohen Freue GV, Oosthuizen JL, Kam SH, Ruan J, Takhar MK, et al. Plasma proteomics can discriminate isolated early from dual responses in asthmatic individuals undergoing an allergen inhalation challenge. Proteomics Clin Appl. 2012;6(9–10):476–85.

306. Izbicka E, Streeper RT, Michalek JE, Louden CL, Diaz A 3rd, Campos DR. Plasma biomarkers distinguish non-small cell lung cancer from asthma and differ in men and women. Cancer Genomics Proteomics. 2012;9(1):27–35.

307. Verrills NM, Irwin JA, He XY, Wood LG, Powell H, Simpson JL, et al. Identification of novel diagnostic biomarkers for asthma and chronic obstructive pulmonary disease. Am J Respir Crit Care Med. 2011;183(12):1633–43.

308. Araújo L, Moreira A, Palmares C, Beltrão M, Fonseca J, Delgado L. Induced sputum in children: success determinants, safety, and cell profiles. J Investig Allergol Clin Immunol. 2011;21(3):216–21.

309. Dasgupta A, Nair P. When are biomarkers useful in the management of airway diseases? Pol Arch Med Wewn. 2013;123(4):183–8.

310. Efthimiadis A, Spanevello A, Hamid Q, Kelly MM, Linden M, Louis R, et al. Methods of sputum processing for cell counts, immunocytochemistry and in situ hybridisation. Eur Respir J Suppl. 2002;37:19s–23s.

311. Gershman NH, Wong HH, Liu JT, Mahlmeister MJ, Fahy JV. Comparison of two methods of collecting induced sputum in asthmatic subjects. Eur Respir J. 1996;9(12):2448–53.

312. Pin I, Gibson PG, Kolendowicz R, Girgis-Gabardo A, Denburg JA, Hargreave FE, et al. Use of induced sputum cell counts to investigate airway inflammation in asthma. Thorax. 1992;47(1):25–9.

313. Pizzichini E, Pizzichini MM, Efthimiadis A, Hargreave FE, Dolovich J. Measurement of inflammatory indices in induced sputum: effects of

selection of sputum to minimize salivary contamination. Eur Respir J. 1996;9(6):1174–80.

314. Fireman E, Toledano B, Buchner N, Stark M, Schwarz Y. Simplified detection of eosinophils in induced sputum. Inflamm Res. 2011;60(8):745–50.

315. Goncalves J, Pizzichini E, Pizzichini MM, Steidle LJ, Rocha CC, Ferreira SC, et al. Reliability of a rapid hematology stain for sputum cytology. J Bras Pneumol. 2014;40(3):250–8.

316. Wenzel SE, Schwartz LB, Langmack EL, Halliday JL, Trudeau JB, Gibbs RL, et al. Evidence that severe asthma can be divided pathologically into two inflammatory subtypes with distinct physiologic and clinical characteristics. Am J Respir Crit Care Med. 1999;160(3):1001–8.

317. Simpson JL, Scott R, Boyle MJ, Gibson PG. Inflammatory subtypes in asthma: assessment and identification using induced sputum. Respirology. 2006;11(1):54–61.

318. Reddel HK, Taylor DR, Bateman ED, Boulet LP, Boushey HA, Busse WW, et al. An official American Thoracic Society/European Respiratory Society statement: asthma control and exacerbations: standardizing endpoints for clinical asthma trials and clinical practice. Am J Respir Crit Care Med. 2009;180(1):59–99.

319. Belda J, Leigh R, Parameswaran K, O'Byrne PM, Sears MR, Hargreave FE. Induced sputum cell counts in healthy adults. Am J Respir Crit Care Med. 2000;161(2 Pt 1):475–8.

320. Louis R, Sele J, Henket M, Cataldo D, Bettiol J, Seiden L, et al. Sputum eosinophil count in a large population of patients with mild to moderate steroid-naive asthma: distribution and relationship with methacholine bronchial hyperresponsiveness. Allergy. 2002;57(10):907–12.

321. in't Veen JC, Smits HH, Hiemstra PS, Zwinderman AE, Sterk PJ, Bel EH. Lung function and sputum characteristics of patients with severe asthma during an induced exacerbation by double-blind steroid withdrawal. Am J Respir Crit Care Med. 1999;160(1):93–9.

322. Hastie AT, Moore WC, Meyers DA, Vestal PL, Li H, Peters SP, et al. Analyses of asthma severity phenotypes and inflammatory proteins in subjects stratified by sputum granulocytes. J Allergy Clin Immunol. 2010;125(5):1028–36. e13

323. Jatakanon A, Lim S, Barnes PJ. Changes in sputum eosinophils predict loss of asthma control. Am J Respir Crit Care Med. 2000;161(1):64–72.

324. Woodruff PG, Khashayar R, Lazarus SC, Janson S, Avila P, Boushey HA, et al. Relationship between airway inflammation, hyperresponsiveness, and obstruction in asthma. J Allergy Clin Immunol. 2001;108(5):753–8.

325. Berry M, Morgan A, Shaw DE, Parker D, Green R, Brightling C, et al. Pathological features and inhaled corticosteroid response of eosinophilic and non-eosinophilic asthma. Thorax. 2007;62(12):1043–9.

326. Green RH, Brightling CE, Woltmann G, Parker D, Wardlaw AJ, Pavord ID. Analysis of induced sputum in adults with asthma: identification of subgroup with isolated sputum neutrophilia and poor response to inhaled corticosteroids. Thorax. 2002;57(10):875–9.

327. Green RH, Brightling CE, McKenna S, Hargadon B, Parker D, Bradding P, et al. Asthma exacerbations and sputum eosinophil counts: a randomised controlled trial. Lancet. 2002;360(9347):1715–21.

328. van Rensen EL, Straathof KC, Veselic-Charvat MA, Zwinderman AH, Bel EH, Sterk PJ. Effect of inhaled steroids on airway hyperresponsiveness, sputum eosinophils, and exhaled nitric oxide levels in patients with asthma. Thorax. 1999;54(5):403–8.

329. Pizzichini MM, Pizzichini E, Clelland L, Efthimiadis A, Mahony J, Dolovich J, et al. Sputum in severe exacerbations of asthma: kinetics of inflammatory indices after prednisone treatment. Am J Respir Crit Care Med. 1997;155(5):1501–8.

330. Leuppi JD, Salome CM, Jenkins CR, Anderson SD, Xuan W, Marks GB, et al. Predictive markers of asthma exacerbation during stepwise dose reduction of inhaled corticosteroids. Am J Respir Crit Care Med. 2001;163(2):406–12.

331. Deykin A, Lazarus SC, Fahy JV, Wechsler ME, Boushey HA, Chinchilli VM, et al. Sputum eosinophil counts predict asthma control after discontinuation of inhaled corticosteroids. J Allergy Clin Immunol. 2005;115(4):720–7.

332. Flood-Page P, Swenson C, Faiferman I, Matthews J, Williams M, Brannick L, et al. A study to evaluate safety and efficacy of mepolizumab in patients with moderate persistent asthma. Am J Respir Crit Care Med. 2007;176(11):1062–71.

333. Moore WC, Hastie AT, Li X, Li H, Busse WW, Jarjour NN, et al. Sputum neutrophil counts are associated with more severe asthma phenotypes using cluster analysis. J Allergy Clin Immunol. 2014;133(6):1557–63.e5.

334. Wenzel SE, Szefler SJ, Leung DY, Sloan SI, Rex MD, Martin RJ. Bronchoscopic evaluation of severe asthma. Persistent inflammation associated with high dose glucocorticoids. Am J Respir Crit Care Med. 1997;156(3 Pt 1):737–43.

335. Choi JS, Jang AS, Park JS, Park SW, Paik SH, Park JS, et al. Role of neutrophils in persistent airway obstruction due to refractory asthma. Respirology. 2012;17(2):322–9.

336. Schleich FN, Manise M, Sele J, Henket M, Seidel L, Louis R. Distribution of sputum cellular phenotype in a large asthma cohort: predicting factors for eosinophilic vs neutrophilic inflammation. BMC Pulm Med. 2013;13:11.

337. Cowan DC, Cowan JO, Palmay R, Williamson A, Taylor DR. Effects of steroid therapy on inflammatory cell subtypes in asthma. Thorax. 2010;65(5):384–90.

338. Nguyen LT, Lim S, Oates T, Chung KF. Increase in airway neutrophils after oral but not inhaled

corticosteroid therapy in mild asthma. Respir Med. 2005;99(2):200–7.

339. Shannon J, Ernst P, Yamauchi Y, Olivenstein R, Lemiere C, Foley S, et al. Differences in airway cytokine profile in severe asthma compared to moderate asthma. Chest. 2008;133(2):420–6.

340. McKinley L, Alcorn JF, Peterson A, Dupont RB, Kapadia S, Logar A, et al. TH17 cells mediate steroid-resistant airway inflammation and airway hyperresponsiveness in mice. J Immunol. 2008;181(6):4089–97.

341. Al-Ramli W, Prefontaine D, Chouiali F, Martin JG, Olivenstein R, Lemiere C, et al. T(H)17-associated cytokines (IL-17A and IL-17F) in severe asthma. J Allergy Clin Immunol. 2009;123(5):1185–7.

342. Lajoie S, Lewkowich IP, Suzuki Y, Clark JR, Sproles AA, Dienger K, et al. Complement-mediated regulation of the IL-17A axis is a central genetic determinant of the severity of experimental allergic asthma. Nat Immunol. 2010;11(10):928–35.

343. Hastie AT, Moore WC, Li H, Rector BM, Ortega VE, Pascual RM, et al. Biomarker surrogates do not accurately predict sputum eosinophil and neutrophil percentages in asthmatic subjects. J Allergy Clin Immunol. 2013;132(1):72–80.

344. Bakakos P, Schleich F, Alchanatis M, Louis R. Induced sputum in asthma: from bench to bedside. Curr Med Chem. 2011;18(10):1415–22.

345. Koh GC, Shek LP, Goh DY, Van Bever H, Koh DS. Eosinophil cationic protein: is it useful in asthma? A systematic review. Respir Med. 2007;101(4):696–705.

346. Kim CK, Callaway Z, Fletcher R, Koh YY. Eosinophil-derived neurotoxin in childhood asthma: correlation with disease severity. J Asthma. 2010;47(5):568–73.

347. Pavord ID, Bafadhel M. Exhaled nitric oxide and blood eosinophilia: independent markers of preventable risk. J Allergy Clin Immunol. 2013;132(4):828–9.

348. Jia CE, Zhang HP, Lv Y, Liang R, Jiang YQ, Powell H, et al. The Asthma Control Test and Asthma Control Questionnaire for assessing asthma control: systematic review and meta-analysis. J Allergy Clin Immunol. 2013;131(3):695–703.

349. Mostafa GA, Reda SM, Abd El-Aziz MM, Ahmed SA. Sputum neurokinin A in Egyptian asthmatic children and adolescents: relation to exacerbation severity. Allergy. 2008;63(9):1244–7.

350. Yamaguchi M, Niimi A, Matsumoto H, Ueda T, Takemura M, Matsuoka H, et al. Sputum levels of transforming growth factor-beta1 in asthma: relation to clinical and computed tomography findings. J Investig Allergol Clin Immunol. 2008;18(3):202–6.

351. Mattos W, Lim S, Russell R, Jatakanon A, Chung KF, Barnes PJ. Matrix metalloproteinase-9 expression in asthma: effect of asthma severity, allergen challenge, and inhaled corticosteroids. Chest. 2002;122(5):1543–52.

352. Saito J, Zhang Q, Hui C, Macedo P, Gibeon D, Menzies-Gow A, et al. Sputum hydrogen sulfide as a novel biomarker of obstructive neutrophilic asthma. J Allergy Clin Immunol. 2013;131(1):232–4 e1-3.

353. Brickey WJ, Alexis NE, Hernandez ML, Reed W, Ting JP, Peden DB. Sputum inflammatory cells from patients with allergic rhinitis and asthma have decreased inflammasome gene expression. J Allergy Clin Immunol. 2011;128(4):900–3.

354. Alexis NE, Soukup J, Nierkens S, Becker S. Association between airway hyperreactivity and bronchial macrophage dysfunction in individuals with mild asthma. Am J Physiol Lung Cell Mol Physiol. 2001;280(2):L369–75.

355. Alexis NE, Brickey WJ, Lay JC, Wang Y, Roubey RA, Ting JP, et al. Development of an inhaled endotoxin challenge protocol for characterizing evoked cell surface phenotype and genomic responses of airway cells in allergic individuals. Ann Allergy Asthma Immunol. 2008;100(3):206–15.

356. Loughlin CE, Esther CR Jr, Lazarowski ER, Alexis NE, Peden DB. Neutrophilic inflammation is associated with altered airway hydration in stable asthmatics. Respir Med. 2010;104(1):29–33.

357. Brightling CE, Symon FA, Birring SS, Bradding P, Pavord ID, Wardlaw AJ. TH2 cytokine expression in bronchoalveolar lavage fluid T lymphocytes and bronchial submucosa is a feature of asthma and eosinophilic bronchitis. J Allergy Clin Immunol. 2002;110(6):899–905.

358. Alexis NE, Hu SC, Zeman K, Alter T, Bennett WD. Induced sputum derives from the central airways: confirmation using a radiolabeled aerosol bolus delivery technique. Am J Respir Crit Care Med. 2001;164(10 Pt 1):1964–70.

359. Alexis N, Soukup J, Ghio A, Becker S. Sputum phagocytes from healthy individuals are functional and activated: a flow cytometric comparison with cells in bronchoalveolar lavage and peripheral blood. Clin Immunol. 2000;97(1):21–32.

360. Goleva E, Jackson LP, Harris JK, Robertson CE, Sutherland ER, Hall CF, et al. The effects of airway microbiome on corticosteroid responsiveness in asthma. Am J Respir Crit Care Med. 2013;188(10):1193–201.

361. Esnault S, Kelly EA, Schwantes EA, Liu LY, DeLain LP, Hauer JA, et al. Identification of genes expressed by human airway eosinophils after an in vivo allergen challenge. PLoS One. 2013;8(7):e67560.

362. Vargas JE, Porto BN, Puga R, Stein RT, Pitrez PM. Identifying a biomarker network for corticosteroid resistance in asthma from bronchoalveolar lavage samples. Mol Biol Rep. 2016;43(7):697–710.

363. Park SW, Lee EH, Lee EJ, Kim HJ, Bae DJ, Han S, et al. Apolipoprotein A1 potentiates lipoxin A4 synthesis and recovery of allergen-induced disrupted tight junctions in the airway epithelium. Clin Exp Allergy. 2013;43(8):914–27.

364. Sampson AP. The leukotrienes: mediators of chronic inflammation in asthma. Clin Exp Allergy. 1996;26(9):995–1004.

365. Montuschi P, Peters-Golden ML. Leukotriene modifiers for asthma treatment. Clin Exp Allergy. 2010;40(12):1732–41.

366. Montuschi P, Santini G, Valente S, Mondino C, Macagno F, Cattani P, et al. Liquid chromatography-mass spectrometry measurement of leukotrienes in asthma and other respiratory diseases. J Chromatogr B. 2014;964:12–25.

367. Severien C, Artlich A, Jonas S, Becher G. Urinary excretion of leukotriene E4 and eosinophil protein X in children with atopic asthma. Eur Respir J. 2000;16(4):588–92.

368. Suzuki N, Hishinuma T, Abe F, Omata K, Ito S, Sugiyama M, et al. Difference in urinary LTE4 and 11-dehydro-TXB2 excretion in asthmatic patients. Prostaglandins Other Lipid Mediat. 2000;62(4):395–403.

369. Aggarwal S, Moodley YP, Thompson PJ, Misso NL. Prostaglandin E2 and cysteinyl leukotriene concentrations in sputum: association with asthma severity and eosinophilic inflammation. Clin Exp Allergy. 2010;40(1):85–93.

370. Marmarinos A, Saxoni-Papageorgiou P, Cassimos D, Manoussakis E, Tsentidis C, Doxara A, et al. Urinary leukotriene E4 levels in atopic and non-atopic preschool children with recurrent episodic (viral) wheezing: a potential marker? J Asthma. 2015;52(6):554–9.

371. Morales M, Flores C, Pino K, Angulo J, Lopez-Lastra M, Castro-Rodriguez JA. Urinary leukotriene and Bcl I polymorphism of glucocorticoid receptor gene in preschoolers with recurrent wheezing and high risk of asthma. Allergol Immunopathol. 2016;44(1):59–65.

372. Chiu CY, Tsai MH, Yao TC, Tu YL, Hua MC, Yeh KW, et al. Urinary LTE4 levels as a diagnostic marker for IgE-mediated asthma in preschool children: a birth cohort study. PLoS One. 2014;9(12):e115216.

373. Higashi N, Mita H, Ono E, Fukutomi Y, Yamaguchi H, Kajiwara K, et al. Profile of eicosanoid generation in aspirin-intolerant asthma and anaphylaxis assessed by new biomarkers. J Allergy Clin Immunol. 2010;125(5):1084–91. e6

374. O'Shaughnessy KM, Wellings R, Gillies B, Fuller RW. Differential effects of fluticasone propionate on allergen-evoked bronchoconstriction and increased urinary leukotriene E4 excretion. Am Rev Respir Dis. 1993;147(6 Pt 1):1472–6.

375. Liu MC, Dube LM, Lancaster J. Acute and chronic effects of a 5-lipoxygenase inhibitor in asthma: a 6-month randomized multicenter trial. Zileuton Study Group. J Allergy Clin Immunol. 1996;98(5 Pt 1):859–71.

376. Thomson NC, Chaudhuri R, Spears M, Messow CM, Jelinsky S, Miele G, et al. Arachidonic acid metabolites and enzyme transcripts in asthma are altered by cigarette smoking. Allergy. 2014;69(4):527–36.

377. Rabinovitch N, Reisdorph N, Silveira L, Gelfand EW. Urinary leukotriene E(4) levels identify children with tobacco smoke exposure at risk for asthma exacerbation. J Allergy Clin Immunol. 2011;128(2):323–7.

378. Murray JJ, Tonnel AB, Brash AR, Roberts LJ 2nd, Gosset P, Workman R, et al. Release of prostaglandin D2 into human airways during acute antigen challenge. N Engl J Med. 1986;315(13):800–4.

379. O'Sullivan S, Dahlen B, Dahlen SE, Kumlin M. Increased urinary excretion of the prostaglandin D2 metabolite 9 alpha, 11 beta-prostaglandin F2 after aspirin challenge supports mast cell activation in aspirin-induced airway obstruction. J Allergy Clin Immunol. 1996;98(2):421–32.

380. Nagakura T, Obata T, Shichijo K, Matsuda S, Sigimoto H, Yamashita K, et al. GC/MS analysis of urinary excretion of 9alpha,11beta-PGF2 in acute and exercise-induced asthma in children. Clin Exp Allergy. 1998;28(2):181–6.

381. Misso NL, Aggarwal S, Phelps S, Beard R, Thompson PJ. Urinary leukotriene E4 and 9 alpha, 11 beta-prostaglandin F concentrations in mild, moderate and severe asthma, and in healthy subjects. Clin Exp Allergy. 2004;34(4):624–31.

382. Reimert CM, Minuva U, Kharazmi A, Bendtzen K. Eosinophil protein X/eosinophil derived neurotoxin (EPX/EDN). Detection by enzyme-linked immunosorbent assay and purification from normal human urine. J Immunol Methods. 1991;141(1):97–104.

383. Klonoff-Cohen H, Polavarapu M. Eosinophil protein X and childhood asthma: a systematic review and meta-analysis. Immun Inflamm Dis. 2016;4(2):114–34.

384. Khalil Kalaajieh W, Hoilat R. Asthma attack severity and urinary concentration of eosinophil X protein in children. Allergol Immunopathol. 2002;30(4):225–31.

385. Nuijsink M, Hop WC, Sterk PJ, Duiverman EJ, De Jongste JC. Urinary eosinophil protein X in childhood asthma: relation with changes in disease control and eosinophilic airway inflammation. Mediat Inflamm. 2013;2013:532619.

386. Wu W, Chen Y, d'Avignon A, Hazen SL. 3-Bromotyrosine and 3,5-dibromotyrosine are major products of protein oxidation by eosinophil peroxidase: potential markers for eosinophil-dependent tissue injury in vivo. Biochemistry. 1999;38(12):3538–48.

387. Wu W, Samoszuk MK, Comhair SA, Thomassen MJ, Farver CF, Dweik RA, et al. Eosinophils generate brominating oxidants in allergen-induced asthma. J Clin Invest. 2000;105(10):1455–63.

388. Wedes SH, Wu W, Comhair SA, McDowell KM, DiDonato JA, Erzurum SC, et al. Urinary bromotyrosine measures asthma control and predicts asthma exacerbations in children. J Pediatr. 2011;159(2):248–55.

Radiologic Diagnostic Modalities in Severe Asthma

Gong Yong Jin

Asthma is a chronic inflammatory disease of the airways. Chronic inflammation is present in almost all patients with asthma, even in the airways of patients with very mild asthma, and increases with disease severity. Asthma affects approximately 5% of the general adult population, of whom approximately 5–10% suffer from severe asthma [1].

Long-standing severe asthma may be associated with structural changes of both the proximal and distal airways. Pulmonary function studies are the main measures used to assess and monitor airway obstruction in asthma. Although the significance of radiological findings of asthma remains unclear, high-resolution CT (HRCT) scan has identified abnormalities in asthma and has correlated these abnormalities with clinical and pulmonary function data. In severe asthma, the applications of HRCT scanning are considerably broader. This technique has been used to noninvasively assess airway wall changes in patients with severe asthma. Over the past 10 years, HRCT scan has been validated as an appropriate technique for distinguishing patients with asthma with normal airflow or mild airflow obstruction from healthy subjects [2–5].

HRCT scan has enabled visualization of airways and parenchyma in much greater detail than plain radiography. Expected abnormalities were seen in 37.8% of the chest radiographs, while the HRCT scans were abnormal in 71.9% of the cases. Pathologically, the structural changes in severe asthma comprise bronchiectasis with mucoid impaction, bronchial dilatation, and bronchial wall thickening (Fig. 5.1), although some causes of wall thickening such as airway wall edema, mucoid impaction, and bronchoconstriction are potentially reversible [6]. Inspiratory HRCT findings in subjects with asthma are identical to abnormal radiologic findings, such as bronchial wall thickening (BWT), bronchial wall dilatation, bronchiectasis (BE), mosaic lung

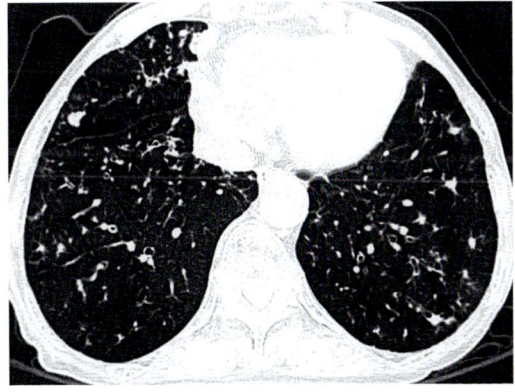

Fig. 5.1 Images from a 78/F subject who was diagnosed with bronchial asthma 5 years ago. The HRCT scans show diffuse bronchial wall thickening with dilatation, mucoid retention, and a mosaic pattern in both lower lobes

G.Y. Jin
Department of Radiology, Chonbuk National University Medical School,
Jeonju 54907, South Korea
e-mail: gyjin@chonbuk.ac.kr

© Springer Nature Singapore Pte Ltd. 2018
Y.C. Lee et al. (eds.), *Severe Asthma*, https://doi.org/10.1007/978-981-10-1998-2_5

attenuation, mucus plugging, prominent centri-lobular opacities, emphysema, and atelectasis (Table 5.1) [6–8]. Gupta reported that abnormal HRCT scan findings were common in patients with severe asthma (bronchiectasis and bronchial wall thickening were observed in 40% and 62% of all cases, respectively), whereas HRCT scans were normal in only 20% of all cases [9]. More recent studies of the airway immunopathology of asthma have revealed that there is an important chronic inflammatory component characterized by cellular infiltration with eosinophils and lymphocytes, epithelial shedding, and subepithelial fibrosis in the proximal large airways. Extensive inflammatory changes have been noted in the distal airways, which are associated with mucus plugging and airway obstruction or obliteration, in the lungs of patients who died of acute severe asthma [10]. In one group of patients with severe asthma, intrapulmonary airway abnormalities (bronchial dilatation and bronchial thickening) were observed on the HRCT scans of up to 50% of all examined patients [6, 10].

In severe asthma, the small airways are also affected by significant inflammation and remodeling. Small airway dysfunction reduces ventilation in part of the lung, thereby inducing reflex vasoconstriction. This phenomenon is visualized as an area of decreased attenuation on the HRCT images. Heterogeneity of lung attenuation on inspiration CT scans is accentuated in expiratory scans due to regional differences in small airway closure (mosaic perfusion and gas trapping). Therefore, expiratory HRCT has been proposed to be helpful for accessing air trapping (defined as areas of increased lucency on expiratory scans) in severe asthma [11] (Fig. 5.2). The degree of air trapping, together with the reduction in the cross-

Table 5.1 HRCT findings in patients with severe bronchial asthma

Bronchial wall thickening

Cylindrical bronchiectasis

Mucoid impaction in the large bronchi

Thick linear opacity or small centrilobular opacities

Areas of decreased attenuation

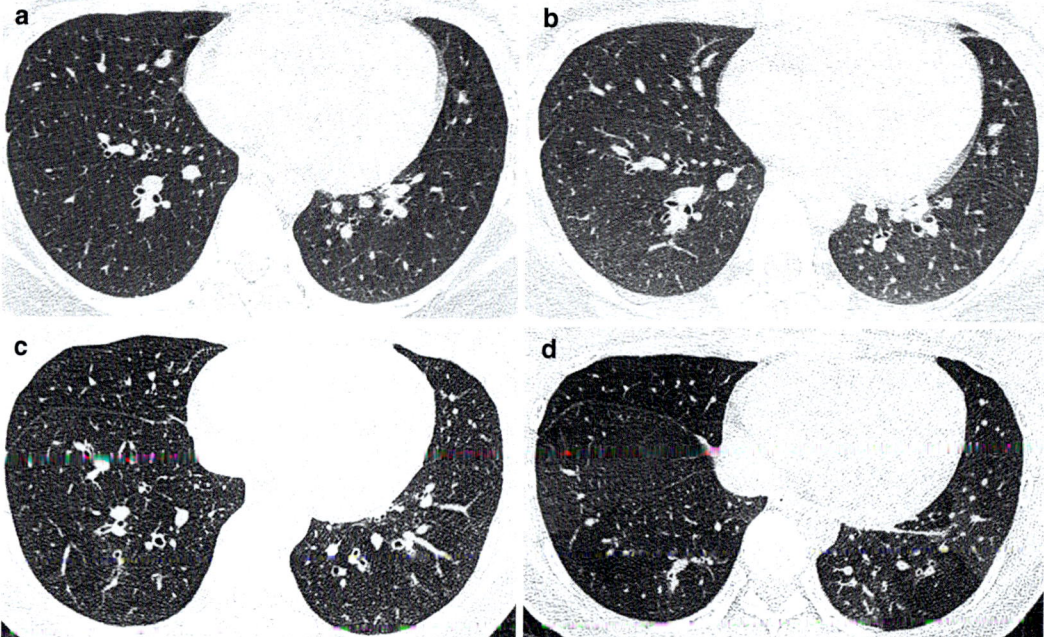

Fig. 5.2 Images from a 30/F patient. (**a**, **b**) Ten years ago, she was diagnosed with bronchial asthma, and her HRCT scans showed nonspecific findings. (**c**, **d**) Ten years later, her HRCT scans showed mild diffuse bronchial wall thickening on inhalation and progressed air trapping on exhalation. The number and size of the blood vessels were both decreased in areas of reduced attenuation. On admission day, her FEV_1 was 0.81 L

sectional area on expiration, has been shown to correlate well with forced expiratory volume in 1 second (FEV_1), indicating that these abnormalities could reflect the severity of asthma. These abnormalities also represent radiological evidence for distal airway obstruction in asthma. In contrast, changes in bronchial dilatation and wall thickening were not significantly correlated with FEV_1 [10, 12]. It is possible that the extent of distal airway obstruction is a feature of severe asthma. In a study by Lynch and colleagues [13], full inspiratory CT scans were acquired from a group of 48 patients with less severe asthma with a mean FEV_1 (% predicted) of 64%. Ten patients showed patchy ($n = 7$) or diffuse ($n = 3$) areas of hyperlucency, which could represent air trapping. Because the distal airways of patients with asthma are not readily accessible for study from either the pathological or physiological point of view, HRCT scan may be a suitable noninvasive method for assessing distal airways. Carr et al. performed inspiratory and expiratory HRCT scans on 24 patients with chronic severe asthma [10]. They observed concomitant dilatation and thickening of the intrapulmonary airways in 12 patients, whereas air trapping was noted in 20 patients. The mean expiratory-to-inspiratory cross-sectional area (Exp/Ins) was 75.9 ± 2.0%, compared with 44.6 ± 1.0% in non-asthmatic subjects. The FEV_1 (% predicted) correlated with the Exp/Ins ratio and with the CT features of air trapping (both $r = 0.60$; $P < 0.001$), but not with airway dilatation or thickening. Peripheral airway obstruction may be common in chronic severe asthma, which may explain the increased severity of this type of asthma.

HRCT assessment of air trapping in asthma has been associated with airway hyperresponsiveness, disease duration, and airflow limitation. This technique has been used to evaluate the response to inhaled steroids. In addition, air trapping has been shown to correlate with asthma severity. The air trapping percentage of patients with severe asthma has been shown to be significantly increased compared with that of normal subjects ($P < 0.005$) [14, 15]. This result was supported by an analysis of tissue fractions at functional residual capacity in patients with severe asthma, which revealed that the fractions are much smaller than in normal subjects on both the dorsal-ventral and basal-apical axes. In addition to the overall air trapping percentage, the lobar distributions of air trapping fractions at functional residual capacity are different between normal subjects and patients with severe asthma. More specifically, the air trapping fractions in the lower lobes of patients with severe asthma are generally increased compared with those of normal subjects [16]. Moreover, the tissue fractions of patients with severe asthma are much smaller than those of normal subjects in the gravitational-dependent and basal regions, implying the presence of air trapping and reduced air volume change. These results are qualitatively consistent with studies of ventilation defects.

In one study, airway abnormalities (bronchial dilatation and bronchial thickening) were observed by HRCT in up to 50% of all patients with severe asthma [6]. Moreover, the airways of patients who die from asthma have thickened walls. Dunnill et al. reported that bronchial smooth muscle accounted for 4.6 + 2.2% of the volume of the normal bronchial wall [17]. However, the volume in patients dying of status asthmaticus was significantly increased, with a mean value of 11.9 + 3.36% [17, 18]. Okazawa and colleagues showed that even small airways (1.5–6 mm luminal diameter) of patients with asthma were significantly thickened compared with those of normal controls [19]. Also, the mean percentages of wall area (WA%) in asthma patients were 84% for small airways (luminal diameter <2 mm) and 58% for large airways (luminal diameter >6 mm). Also, Awadh and colleagues reported that the mean WA% for all airways assessed was 78% for patients with near-fatal asthma but 70.9% for normal controls [18]. Although the predominant site of airway narrowing in asthma is not clear, thickening of the airway wall in patients with fatal asthma was observed in both large cartilaginous and small membranous bronchi. However, this thickening occurred predominantly in the small airways of patients with nonfatal asthma [18, 19]. Gupta et al. reported the RB-proximal third-generation airway was remodeled in patients with severe asthma, with luminal narrowing and an increased WA% [9]. Importantly, WA% was associated with lung function impairment and was significantly greater in patients with severe asthma with persistent airflow obstruction than in those without. Also, WA% has been shown to be associated with the burden of neutrophilic airway inflammation over time, suggesting that this component of the airway inflammatory profile may be important in airway remodeling.

The relationship of airway wall thickening in asthma to lung function remains unclear. FEV_1 in chronic asthma does not appear to reflect bronchial wall thickness as assessed by HRCT scan [20]. Radiologically, observable wall thickening encompasses smooth muscle hyperplasia/hypertrophy and subepithelial fibrosis; extracellular matrix changes and structural changes in one of these locations may be more influential. The subsequent effects on airway mechanics remain unclear, although thickening of the subepithelial layer has been shown to decrease the airway luminal area and exacerbate the effect of airway smooth muscle shortening [20, 21]. In pulmonary function tests, FEF_{25-75} values suggest that small airway function may be influenced more by bronchial wall thickening than by FEV_1. Abnormal HRCT findings [e.g., bronchiectasis (17.5%), emphysema (5.3%), and mosaic pattern of lung attenuation (17.5%)] were more common

in patients with bronchial asthma with moderate to severe airflow limitation (FEV_1 <80%, $P < 0.05$); moreover, patients with these changes had a more prolonged history of asthma ($P < 0.05$) [22].

The focus of the National Institutes of Health (NIH)-sponsored multicenter Severe Asthma Research Program (SARP) is to identify phenotypes enabling the separation of patients with non-severe asthma from patients with severe asthma [23–25]. This search for phenotypes has included the acquisition of volumetric computed tomography (CT) scans of the lungs at both total lung capacity (TLC) and functional residual capacity (FRC) [26]. Quantitative computed tomography (QCT) has emerged as a reliable, noninvasive tool for the assessment of proximal airway remodeling and air trapping in asthma [26]. Airway lumen narrowing is another characteristic of proximal airway morphology in patients with severe asthma, as demonstrated by QCT assessment (Fig. 5.3). In normal subjects, air volume changes, volume change, and anisotropic deformation of the lower lobes are greater than those of subjects with severe asthma. As a result, the dependence of air volume change on the lower lobes is greater than on the upper lobes. In contrast, deformation of the lower lobes is limited in subjects with severe asthma, as suggested by the observed decreased volume change and

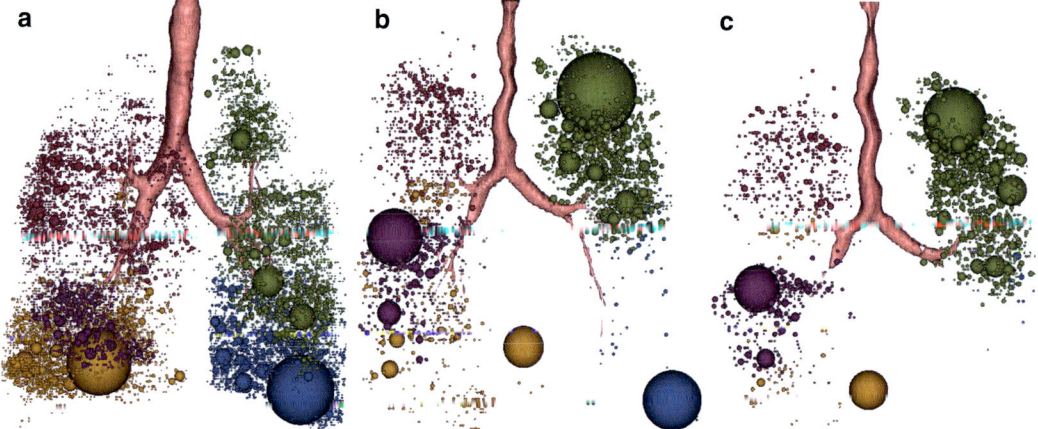

Fig. 5.3 Images of a normal subject (**a**) and a subject with severe bronchial asthma (**b, c**). (**a**) Volume rendering image on a volumetric CT scan of a normal subject. (**b, c**) Images of a 90/F subject who was diagnosed with bron-chial asthma 45 years ago. On admission day, her FEV_1 was 0.037 L. The volume rendering image on the volumetric CT scan shows severe airway remodeling on inspiration and expiration

reduced anisotropic deformation. These changes result in increased volume change and enhanced anisotropic deformation in the upper lobes [26]. In both normal subjects and subjects with severe asthma, CT-based total lung volume (CT) and air volume (CT) are significantly correlated with PFT-based volumes at both TLC and FRC. In addition, the TLVs (CT) are in similar ranges (~90%) as the PFT volumes [26, 27]. For air volume (CT), approximately 20% and 40% reductions from PFTs are measured at TLC and FRC, respectively, in both normal subjects and subjects with severe asthma [28]. The air volume change in normal lungs increases gradually from the apex to the base (from 20% to 80%) and from the ventral to dorsal lung regions, whereas air volume becomes fairly uniformly distributed in subjects with severe asthma. Furthermore, the air volume change and volume change in subjects with severe asthma are increased in the upper lobes but decreased in the lower lobes compared with normal subjects. Accordingly, the reduced air volume change in subjects with severe asthma occurs mainly in the lower lobes. This idea is supported by analyses comparing the contours of air volume change that captured nearly 80% of the apical-to-basal distance [29].

Advances in CT technology and post-processing software have quantitative assessments of the airway tree and the lung parenchyma [9, 26, 29, 30]. Multi-detector row CT scanners facilitate isotropic acquisition of the whole chest with submillimeter resolution within a single breath-hold. Furthermore, rapid advances in post-processing software for CT images now permit multi-planar reconstructions, acquisition of three-dimensional surface and volume images of the airway tree and lung parenchyma, detailed quantitative analysis, and virtual bronchoscopy. Quantitative imaging techniques have enabled us to obtain direct measurements by three-dimensional assessment of the large airways, as well as by indirect assessment of the small airways by densitometric measures of paired inspiratory and expiratory scans. Exact measurement of the airway wall, which requires identification of the lumen-wall and wall-parenchyma boundaries on CT images, is still an inexact sci-ence. However, a number of algorithms have been proposed. One of the earliest proposed techniques is the "full width at half maximum" principle [12, 31]. Although this technique is the most widely used technique at present, it can cause systematic errors in airway wall and lumen estimation due to the blurring of edges by the CT scanner's point spread function, the oblique orientation of the airways, the algorithm used for image reconstruction, and/or the size of the analyzed airway [12]. To overcome these problems, various methods have been developed, including the "Laplacian and Gaussian" algorithm [13], which utilizes smoothing and edge detection filters to segment airways; the "integral-based method," which minimizes the CT scanner's blurring effect; and the "phase congruency method," which uses multiple reconstruction algorithms to localize the airway wall. However, most of these new software platforms were designed for volumetric CT scans, not for standard HRCT scans. This aspect limits their application to retrospective analysis of archived scans [26].

In the early 1970s, Chiro et al. introduced the concept of dual-energy CT (DECT) [32]. Xenon-enhanced DECT is a novel modality for evaluating regional lung ventilation function. When combined with the dual-energy technique, xenon ventilation CT can reveal normal pulmonary ventilation and is also technically feasible for dynamic or static evaluation of regional ventilation in asthma. Chae et al. analyzed 22 patients with stable asthma by xenon-enhanced DECT and found that patients with asthma with ventilation defects had more severe airflow limitation and airway wall thickening [33]. They also found that patients with asthma with ventilation defects had a lower FEV_1 and that the ventilation defect score was negatively correlated with FEV_1/FVC and the corrected diffusing capacity. Since xenon-enhanced DECT has several limitations (e.g., high radiation exposure, side effects of xenon gas inhalation, and high cost), DECT ventilation imaging with inhaled administration of xenon has been investigated at fewer centers than other imaging techniques [34, 35].

Functional images of ventilation using hyper-polarized helium-3 magnetic resonance imaging

(H³HeMRI) have also been used extensively in studies of subjects with asthma [36]. Patterns of hyperpolarized He-3 gas signal distribution tend to change dynamically within a single breath-hold. Regional changes of airflow obstruction in subjects with asthma observable by H³HeMRI have been shown to correlate with measures of asthma severity and spirometry. Specifically, the rate at which voxel signals show the trend toward a more homogeneous pattern differs by asthma severity. The fastest rate of change was observed in subjects with mild-to-moderate asthma, while otherwise healthy subjects with severe asthma showed relatively slow (yet statistically equivalent) rates of change. These findings were surprising, considering that subjects with severe asthma subjects had the greatest overall spatial heterogeneity in ventilation upon breath-hold initiation at end-inhalation [37].

In conclusion, severe asthma is a complex heterogeneous disease with high morbidity and mortality. Nonradiologic assessments fail to reliably predict important bronchial wall changes; therefore, HRCT scan may be beneficial for all patients with severe asthma. HRCT scan is a repeatable and accurate tool for noninvasive assessment of proximal airway structural changes in patients with severe asthma. In addition, quantitative CT is a reliable, noninvasive tool for quantitative assessment of proximal airway remodeling and air trapping in severe asthma. Moreover, airway wall thickness in severe asthma progresses over time, as assessed by robust quantitative measures of wall thickness.

References

1. Bousquet J, Chanez P, Lacoste JY, Barneon G, Ghavanian N, Enander I, et al. Eosinophilic inflammation in asthma. N Engl J Med. 1990;323(15):1033–9.
2. Park CS, Muller NL, Worthy SA, Kim JS, Awadh N, FitzGerald M. Airway obstruction in asthmatic and healthy individuals: inspiratory and expiratory thin-section CT findings. Radiology. 1997;203(2):361–7.
3. Wenzel S. Severe asthma in adults. Am J Respir Crit Care Med. 2005;172(2):149–60.
4. FitzGerald JM, Bateman E, Hurd S, Boulet LP, Haahtela T, Cruz AA, et al. The GINA asthma challenge: reducing asthma hospitalisations. Eur Respir J. 2011;38(5):997–8.
5. Niimi A, Matsumoto H, Takemura M, Ueda T, Nakano Y, Mishima M. Clinical assessment of airway remodeling in asthma: utility of computed tomography. Clin Rev Allergy Immunol. 2004;27(1):45–58.
6. Paganin F, Trussard V, Seneterre E, Chanez P, Giron J, Godard P, et al. Chest radiography and high resolution computed tomography of the lungs in asthma. Am Rev Respir Dis. 1992;146(4):1084–7.
7. Webb WR. High-resolution computed tomography of obstructive lung disease. Radiol Clin N Am. 1994;32(4):745–57.
8. Harmanci E, Kebapci M, Metintas M, Ozkan R. High-resolution computed tomography findings are correlated with disease severity in asthma. Respiration. 2002;69(5):420–6.
9. Gupta S, Siddiqui S, Haldar P, Entwisle JJ, Mawby D, Wardlaw AJ, et al. Quantitative analysis of high-resolution computed tomography scans in severe asthma subphenotypes. Thorax. 2010;65(9):775–81.
10. Carr DH, Hibon S, Rubens M, Chung KF. Peripheral airways obstruction on high-resolution computed tomography in chronic severe asthma. Respir Med. 1998;92(3):448–53.
11. Witt CA, Sheshadri A, Carlstrom L, Tarsi J, Kozlowski J, Wilson B, et al. Longitudinal changes in airway remodeling and air trapping in severe asthma. Acad Radiol. 2014;21(8):986–93.
12. Bumbacea D, Campbell D, Nguyen L, Carr D, Barnes PJ, Robinson D, et al. Parameters associated with persistent airflow obstruction in chronic severe asthma. Eur Respir J. 2004;24(1):122–8.
13. Lynch DA, Newell JD, Tschomper BA, Cink TM, Newman LS, Bethel R. Uncomplicated asthma in adults: comparison of CT appearance of the lungs in asthmatic and healthy subjects. Radiology. 1993;188(3):829–33.
14. Choi S, Hoffman EA, Wenzel SE, Tawhai MH, Yin Y, Castro M, et al. Registration-based assessment of regional lung function via volumetric CT images of normal subjects vs. severe asthmatics. J Appl Physiol (1985). 2013;115(5):730–42.
15. Busacker A, Newell JD Jr, Keefe T, Hoffman EA, Granroth JC, Castro M, et al. A multivariate analysis of risk factors for the air-trapping asthmatic phenotype as measured by quantitative CT analysis. Chest. 2009;135(1):48–56.
16. Fain SB, Gonzalez-Fernandez G, Peterson ET, Evans MD, Sorkness RL, Jarjour NN, et al. Evaluation of structure-function relationships in asthma using multidetector CT and hyperpolarized He-3 MRI. Acad Radiol. 2008;15(6):753–62.
17. Dunnill MS, Massarella GR, Anderson JA. A comparison of the quantitative anatomy of the bronchi in normal subjects, in status asthmaticus, in chronic bronchitis, and in emphysema. Thorax. 1969;24(2):176–9.
18. Awadh N, Muller NL, Park CS, Abboud RT, FitzGerald JM. Airway wall thickness in patients with near fatal asthma and control groups: assessment

with high resolution computed tomographic scanning. Thorax. 1998;53(4):248–53.

19. Okazawa M, Muller N, McNamara AE, Child S, Verburgt L, Pare PD. Human airway narrowing measured using high resolution computed tomography. Am J Respir Crit Care Med. 1996;154(5):1557–62.

20. James AL, Pare PD, Hogg JC. The mechanics of airway narrowing in asthma. Am Rev Respir Dis. 1989;139(1):242–6.

21. Little SA, Sproule MW, Cowan MD, Macleod KJ, Robertson M, Love JG, et al. High resolution computed tomographic assessment of airway wall thickness in chronic asthma: reproducibility and relationship with lung function and severity. Thorax. 2002;57(3):247–53.

22. Park JW, Hong YK, Kim CW, Kim DK, Choe KO, Hong CS. High-resolution computed tomography in patients with bronchial asthma: correlation with clinical features, pulmonary functions and bronchial hyperresponsiveness. J Investig Allergol Clin Immunol. 1997;7(3):186–92.

23. Moore WC, Bleecker ER, Curran-Everett D, Erzurum SC, Ameredes BT, Bacharier L, et al. Characterization of the severe asthma phenotype by the National Heart, Lung, and Blood Institute's Severe Asthma Research Program. J Allergy Clin Immunol. 2007;119(2):405–13.

24. Moore WC, Meyers DA, Wenzel SE, Teague WG, Li H, Li X, et al. Identification of asthma phenotypes using cluster analysis in the Severe Asthma Research Program. Am J Respir Crit Care Med. 2010;181(4):315–23.

25. Jarjour NN, Erzurum SC, Bleecker ER, Calhoun WJ, Castro M, Comhair SA, et al. Severe asthma: lessons learned from the National Heart, Lung, and Blood Institute Severe Asthma Research Program. Am J Respir Crit Care Med. 2012;185(4):356–62.

26. Walker C, Gupta S, Hartley R, Brightling CE. Computed tomography scans in severe asthma: utility and clinical implications. Curr Opin Pulm Med. 2012;18(1):42–7.

27. Brown MS, Kim HJ, Abtin F, Da Costa I, Pais R, Ahmad S, et al. Reproducibility of lung and lobar volume measurements using computed tomography Acad Radiol. 2010;17(3):316–22.

28. Sorkness RL, Bleecker ER, Busse WW, Calhoun WJ, Castro M, Chung KF, et al. Lung function in adults with stable but severe asthma: air trapping and incomplete reversal of obstruction with bronchodilation. J Appl Physiol (1985). 2008;104(2):394–403.

29. Gupta S, Siddiqui S, Haldar P, Raj JV, Entwisle JJ, Wardlaw AJ, et al. Qualitative analysis of high-resolution CT scans in severe asthma. Chest. 2009;136(6):1521–8.

30. de Jong PA, Muller NL, Pare PD, Coxson HO. Computed tomographic imaging of the airways: relationship to structure and function. Eur Respir J. 2005;26(1):140–52.

31. Aysola RS, Hoffman EA, Gierada D, Wenzel S, Cook-Granroth J, Tarsi J, et al. Airway remodeling measured by multidetector CT is increased in severe asthma and correlates with pathology. Chest. 2008;134(6):1183 91.

32. Chiro GD, Brooks RA, Kessler RM, et al. Tissue signatures with dual-energy computed tomography. Radiology. 1979;131:521–3.

33. Chae EJ, Seo JB, Lee J, et al. Xenon ventilation imaging using dual-energy computed tomography in asthmatics: initial experience. Investig Radiol. 2010;45:354–61.

34. Kong X, Sheng HX, Lu GM, Meinel FG, Dyer KT, Schoepf UJ, et al. Xenon-enhanced dual-energy CT lung ventilation imaging: techniques and clinical applications. AJR Am J Roentgenol. 2014;202(2): 309–17.

35. Jung JW, Kwon JW, Kim TW, Lee SH, Kim KM, Kang HR, et al. New insight into the assessment of asthma using xenon ventilation computed tomography. Ann Allergy Asthma Immunol. 2013;111(2):90–5.

36. Altes TA, Powers PL, Knight-Scott J, Rakes G, Platts-Mills TAE, de Lange EE, et al. Hyperpolarized 3He lung ventilation imaging in asthmatics: preliminary findings. J Magn Reson Imaging. 2001;13:378–84.

37. Hahn AD, Cadman RV, Sorkness RL, Jarjour NN, Nagle SK, Fain SB. Redistribution of inhaled hyperpolarized 3He gas during breath-hold differs by asthma severity. J Appl Physiol. 2016;120(5): 526–36.

Part IV

Current and Future Therapies for Severe Asthma

Pharmacologic Therapies for Severe Asthma

6

So Ri Kim

6.1 Improved Current Medications: Inhaled Corticosteroids (ICS) and Bronchodilators

According to current available clinical management guidelines for asthma, severe asthmatic patients should be treated by highest levels of current pharmacological options which include high-dose ICS with long-acting β2 agonist (LABA), add-on tiotropium, add-on anti-IgE (omalizumab), add-on anti-IL-5 (mepolizumab and reslizumab), and add-on oral corticosteroid (OCS) [1].

6.1.1 Corticosteroids

6.1.1.1 High Dose of ICS or OCS

The list of high-dose ICSs for adult patients is shown in Table 6.1. Some reports have demonstrated that higher dose of ICSs may be more effective in severe asthma than conventional dose of ICS [2, 3]. In addition, several studies have addressed that for moderate-to-severe asthmatic patients, a strategy using budesonide/formoterol

combination inhaler as a reliever is helpful to achieve asthma control and to reduce acute exacerbation [4]. As described above, OCS is often prescribed as maintenance therapy in severe asthma. If so, the physicians want to determine when is optimal to initiate OCS therapy for severe asthmatic patients; however, the correct answer to this question has not been defined. Similarly, it is not yet clear whether continuous low-dose OCS are better than multiple discontinuous bursts for controlling exacerbations. While guidelines for the use of biomarkers to guide CS use have been proposed, the use of sputum eosinophils and/or exhaled nitric oxide levels for guiding therapy in severe asthma remains controversial [5].

6.1.1.2 New ICSs

Since patients with severe asthma might often require high doses of ICSs, the development of new ICS with improving pharmacologic effects and fewer systemic side effects has been expected. Ciclesonide is one of new ICSs and appears to have the least systemic effects and local side effects thanks to the pharmacologic characteristic that the prodrug is activated in the lungs to the active principle des-ciclesonide by esterases, whereas there is little activation in the oropharynx [6]. This pharmacologic merit lets ciclesonide be useful for the treatment of severe asthma that required higher doses of ICS. Moreover, this agent has been developed as a small-particle ICS metered-dose inhaler administered with hydrofluoroalkane (HFA) as a

S.R. Kim
Division of Respiratory Medicine and Allergy,
Department of Internal Medicine, Chonbuk National
University Medical School,
Jeonju 54907, South Korea
e-mail: sori@jbnu.ac.kr

© Springer Nature Singapore Pte Ltd. 2018
Y.C. Lee et al. (eds.), *Severe Asthma*, https://doi.org/10.1007/978-981-10-1998-2_6

Table 6.1 High daily doses of inhaled corticosteroids

Adults and adolescents (≥12 years)	
Drug	Daily dose (mcg)
Beclomethasone dipropionate (CFC)	>1000
Beclomethasone dipropionate (HFA)	>400
Budesonide (DPI)	>800
Ciclesonide (HFA)	>320
Fluticasone furoate (DPI)	200
Fluticasone propionate (DPI)	>500
Fluticasone propionate (HFA)	>500
Mometasone furoate	>440
Triamcinolone acetonide	>2000

propellant. A major advantage of small-particle ICS is that they have improved total lung deposition (i.e., reach to smaller airways), and consequently, effective asthma control is achieved at lower daily doses than the large-particle ICS [7]. Beclomethasone dipropionate is one of new small-particle ICSs. Based on the pharmacologic strengths, we can guess that these new ICSs are more suitable for the treatment of the patient with severe asthma in whom there is inflammation of peripheral airways with evidence of small-airway inflammation [8]. In fact, recent clinical study has demonstrated that patients with persistent airway eosinophilia despite high-dose ICS responded to small-particle formulated ICS, and the use of this new formulated drug targeting the asthmatic group with higher doses of steroid is likely to be beneficial [9].

In addition to particle size of ICS, improving drug half-life may be of interest to some patients with severe asthma. Fluticasone furoate is a newly developed ICS with higher affinity to glucocorticoid receptor leading to improvement of action time compared to previous form of fluticasone, fluticasone propionate [10]. Recent studies with inhaled fluticasone furoate have shown that this translates to enhanced lung residency and once-daily efficacy in asthma [11, 12]. Some evidence has also revealed that the characteristics of fluticasone furoate may result in superior symptom reduction compared with fluticasone propionate [13, 14] or similar improvements in symptoms at less-frequent dosing schedules [15]. In addition, fluticasone furoate was developed as

combination inhaler with LABA, vilanterol for asthmatic patients. A randomized, double-blind, double-dummy, parallel group study has shown that the efficacy of once-daily use of fluticasone furoate/vilanterol was similar to twice-daily fluticasone propionate/salmeterol in improving lung function in patients with persistent uncontrolled asthma [16].

Although ICS is a locally administered drug, not systemic agent, leading to lesser side effects than oral/intravenous corticosteroids, all available ICSs are absorbed from the lungs, and thus they also have the potential for systemic side effects. Many patients are more interested in the harmfulness than their benefits. Based on these unmet needs, dissociated steroid has been developed, which attempts to separate the side effect mechanisms from the anti-inflammatory mechanisms of steroids [17]. Actually, several dissociated steroids have now been developed, including non-glucocorticoid glucocorticoid receptor modulators [18]. However, few have been tested in experimental models of asthma. Only three compounds BI-54903, GW870086X, and AZD5423 have entered clinical development, because it is difficult to uncouple the therapeutic and harmful effects mediated by glucocorticoid receptor unlike the hypothesis and some of the anti-inflammatory effects of corticosteroids might be due to transactivation of anti-inflammatory genes, and therefore selective glucocorticoid receptor activators might not be as efficacious as existing ICSs [18, 19].

6.1.2 LABA

The LABAs have been a major advance in the management of severe asthma and are usually administered through combination inhalers with corticosteroids, since there is convincing evidence that LABAs used without a corticosteroid increase severe exacerbations and mortality. Although there are these concerns about the long-term safety of LABAs in asthmatic patients, new LABAs have been developed for chronic obstructive pulmonary disease (COPD), and these might also reasonably be expected to be effective against

Table 6.2 Ultra long-acting β2 agonists

	Strengths	Selectivity for β_2 over β_1[a]
Indacaterol	Full and potent agonist at β_2-AR[b] and with high intrinsic efficacy A quick onset of action and true 24-h control No antagonism against a short-acting β_2-AR agonist	1.46
Carmoterol	A fast onset and long duration (30 h) of activity	–
Olodaterol	Potent nearly full agonistic response at β_2-AR Low level of β_2-AR desensitization Long duration of action Rapid onset of action comparable to formoterol	2.38
Vilanterol	High β_2 selectivity More rapid onset of activity Significant longer duration of action Low systemic exposure	3.0

[a]Based on $\beta_{1/2/3}$-AR CAMP assays; [b]β_2-adrenoceptor [155]

asthma, specifically as combined formulation with ICS. The recently developed once-daily, very long-acting LABAs are indacaterol, vilanterol, olodaterol, and carmoterol [16, 20–23]. Their chemical properties and clinical strengths of newly developed LABAs are summarized in Table 6.2. Recently, fluticasone furoate/vilanterol and mometasone/indacaterol are developed and used for the asthmatic patients as a combined formulation of new LABAs and ICS. To date, these new ICS/LABA combination therapies to asthmatic patients have shown the comparable or non-inferior efficacy compared to former ICS/LABA treatment in clinical trials [16, 24].

6.1.3 Long-Acting Muscarinic Antagonists (LAMA)

Although LAMA usually was developed and used for COPD patients due to its characteristic that blocks only the cholinergic component of bronchoconstriction resulting in less effectiveness of bronchodilation than β2-agonists which reverse all airway constrictors including the direct effects of inflammatory mediators in asthma, recently its therapeutic indication has been expanded to asthma based on the role of cholinergic pathway or neuronal component in the pathogenesis of asthma. In fact, recent studies have reported that cholinergic activation plays an important role in late response to inhaled allergen in animal models, and muscarinic receptors can

be activated by acetylcholine released from non-neuronal cells, such as epithelial and inflammatory cells [25–27]. Moreover, a representative LAMA, tiotropium, inhibits Th2 cytokine release in allergen-exposed mice and that from human PBMCs [28]. It also reduces eosinophilic inflammation, mucin gene expression, and airway remodeling in a murine model of asthma, possibly through a direct effect on fibroblasts, suggesting that tiotropium might have anti-inflammatory effects through inhibition of acetylcholine action on M3 receptors on inflammatory cells [29]. As for clinical studies, several studies have been performed targeting severe uncontrolled asthma patients to evaluate the effectiveness of LAMA added to ICS alone or ICS/LABA, and the results showed that add-on once-daily tiotropium provided improvement of lung function in some patients of severe asthma and that it has at least comparable pharmacologic effects to salmeterol on bronchodilation in uncontrolled asthma [30–33]. In recent clinical replicate trials, 912 patients with severe asthma were treated with tiotropium as an add-on to high-dose ICS/LABA. Tiotropium significantly improved lung function and asthma control status and increased the time to both the first severe asthma exacerbation and the first episode of asthma worsening [34]. Based on these findings, the recent versions of international guidelines recommend add-on tiotropium as mist formulation to preexisting standard therapy (i.e., high-dose ICS/LABA combination) which is called as triple therapy for severe asthma [1, 35].

In addition to tiotropium, there are several newly developed LAMAs including glycopyrrolate and umeclidinium which are approved bronchodilators for the treatment of COPD, and several clinical trials were identified from recent literature, with ongoing trials listed on www.ClinicalTrials. gov to assess the efficacy of new LAMAs as monotherapy or add-on therapy to ICS alone or ICS/LABA for the patients with asthma [36–38]. The results from the ongoing phase II and phase III studies will help to determine whether new LAMAs may provide an additional option for the treatment of asthma, specifically severe asthma.

6.2 Broad Inflammatory Therapeutic Modalities to Overcome Steroid Resistance

6.2.1 Kinase Inhibitors

Because many kinases are involved in activating the inflammation in asthmatic patients and amplifying the inflammation in severe asthma, this has led to the development of kinase blockers as new anti-inflammatory medicines in asthma [39, 40]. Moreover, several kinases are also associated with the development of steroid resistance through glucocorticoid receptor phosphorylation, enhanced pro-inflammatory gene transcription, or decreased HDAC2 activity [41–45]. In fact, p38 mitogen-activated protein kinase (MAPK) activates inflammatory genes in cells form patients with severe asthma [46]. In addition, activation of MAPK has been found to induce glucocorticoid resistance in inflammatory cells via phosphorylation of glucocorticoid receptor at the site of scrinc 226 [47–49] Many kinds of oral p38 MAPK inhibitors have entered clinical trials for various inflammatory disorders, but none have reached phase III studics because of side effects and toxicity, as well as poor or transient efficacy [50, 51]. The fcasibility of local p38 MAPK inhibition with less systemic side effects has been proved by an experimental data that an inhaled p38 antisense oligonucleotide is effective in suppressing aller-

gic inflammation in mice [52]. Several potent and selective inhaled p38 MAPK inhibitors have been in clinical development for COPD, not yet for asthma [53]. Other MAPKs such as JNK and ERK pathway are also implicated in airway inflammation [54]; however, the selective inhibitors for JNK or ERK are not yet tested in clinical settings of severe asthma [55].

NF-κB is activated in patients with asthma as well as various inflammatory disorders and orchestrates the expression of multiple inflammatory proteins, particularly in patients with severe disease [56, 57]. NF-κB activation is correlated inversely with glucocorticoid responsiveness in patients with severe asthma [44]. Huge amount of evidence has indicated that NF-κB is a potent target of the action mechanism of therapeutic agents for severe asthma including several classic and new antioxidants [58–62]. Interestingly, recent publications have also demonstrated that endoplasmic reticulum (ER) stress is implicated in the pathogenesis of severe asthma through NF-κB signaling pathways, and mitochondrial ROS contributes to induce steroid-resistant asthmatic features via NF-κB activation linked to NLRP3 inflammasome activation in neutrophilic severe asthma animal models [63, 64]. Despite substantial experimental favorable data, there is a big hurdle to develop NF-κB-targeting agents as therapeutics for human disorders due to significant side effects such as immune suppression and defective host defense.

Since pan-phosphoinositide 3-kinase (PI3K) inhibitors (i.e., wortmannin and LY-294002) showed the therapeutic effects on ovalbumin-induced asthmatic features in mice [65], many researchers have been huge interest in defining the role of PI3K and its isoforms in the pathogenesis of bronchial asthma, and enormous knowledge and information on this issue has been gathered. In particular, PI3K-δ activated by oxidative stress may be due to cigarette smoking is implicated in the phosphorylation and inactivation of HDAC2 [45], suggesting that oxidative stress and activation of PI3K-δ signaling might be important mechanisms for steroid resistance in bronchial asthma. Since Lee et al. have, for the first time, reported that PI3K-δ isoform plays a critical role in the pathogenesis of OVA-induced allergic asthma in 2006, enormous amount of studies have revealed the pathogenic role of PI3K isoforms such as δ and/or γ isoforms in various respiratory disorders and the related action mechanisms [66–72]. More interestingly, a recent study has revealed that PI3K-δ isoform regulates fungus-induced steroid-resistant eosinophilic allergic asthmatic inflammation through ER stress [73]. In addition, idelalisib (GS-1101, CAL-101), a potent and selective small-molecule inhibitor of PI3K-δ isoform, appears to reduce allergic responses clinically and immunologically after an environmental allergen challenge in phase I study enrolled with patients with allergic rhinitis which is a representative comorbidity of severe asthma [74]. Consistent with these observations, newly developed PI3K-δ inhibitor as inhaler formulation (GSK2269557) has been tested in clinical trials phase II for asthmatic patients (NCT02567708) and for COPD patients (NCT02294734) with hope that it can be a novel potent therapeutic agent for severe airway disorders.

6.2.2 Antioxidants and Selective Mitochondria-Targeting Antioxidants

The lung is continuously exposed to oxidants, either generated endogenously by metabolic reactions (e.g., from mitochondrial electron transport during respiration or released from phagocytes) or derived from exogenous sources (e.g., air pollutants and cigarette smoke) [75–79]. Recent evidence has supported that increased oxidative stress is related to severity of asthma, propagation of inflammatory response, and reduction of responsiveness to corticosteroids [80]. Actually, under pathologic conditions, oxidative stress exerts a multitude of actions through various signaling pathways involving MAPK, PI3K/Akt, and protein kinase C (PKC), thereby activating pro-inflammatory gene transcription factors such as NF-κB, AP-1, and hypoxia-inducible factor (HIF)-1α [58, 81–89]. Oxidative stress is also involved in production of a number

of inflammatory mediators, most notably eicosanoids, by activating phospholipase A2 (PLA2) [90, 91]. Moreover, oxidative stress also reduces steroid responsiveness through a reduction in HDAC2 activity and expression. Thus, several antioxidants with good bioavailability or molecules that have antioxidant enzyme activity have been developed and tried as therapies through not only protecting against the direct injurious effects of oxidants but also fundamentally altering inflammatory events associated with the pathogenesis of asthma. However, unlike hypothesis and favorable data from animal studies using many antioxidants including N-acetylcysteine (NAC), vitamins C and E, and new generation of antioxidants OTC, AD4, and CB3, previous human studies to evaluate the pharmacologic effects of antioxidants have yielded disappointing results in bronchial asthma so far [54, 58, 61, 62, 85]. Nowadays, mitochondria-targeting antioxidants have been regarded as a breakthrough in antioxidant therapy for severe asthma, since mitochondria is a major source of reactive oxygen species (ROS) in vivo and a promising target organelle for immune and inflammatory responses. In fact, recent studies have revealed that mitochondrial ROS scavenger remarkably attenuated the steroid-resistant asthmatic features which are in both cases associated with not only neutrophilic-dominant inflammation but also eosinophilic-dominant inflammation and TGF-β mediated collagen production in asthma models [63, 73, 92]. In the future, we expect well-designed clinical trials to demonstrate the clinical applicability, safety, and efficacy of these promising therapeutic strategies using antioxidants especially mitochondria-targeting agents for severe asthma.

6.2.3 Phosphodiesterase-4 (PDE4) Inhibitors

Because PDE4 that is a main selective cAMP-metabolizing enzyme is highly expressed in leukocytes and other inflammatory cells involved in the pathogenesis of inflammatory lung diseases, such as asthma and COPD, inhibition of PDE4 has been predicted to have an anti-inflammatory effect and thus therapeutic efficacy [93]. Moreover, in asthma model, PDE4 inhibitor has been reported to show potent anti-inflammatory effects through inhibiting T cells, eosinophils, neutrophils, mast cells, airway smooth muscle, epithelial cells, and nerves [94, 95]. However, the use of PDE4 inhibitor was limited by inconsistent efficacy and significant side effects, in particular gastrointestinal problems such as nausea and vomiting. The only PDE4 inhibitor so far that has demonstrated clinical efficacy with tolerable side effects is roflumilast which is thus the new class of drugs that has gained marketing approval globally for use in patients with severe COPD. Therefore, there has been increased interest in its potential for the treatment of severe asthma [96]. In fact, the effects of PDE4 inhibitors were investigated in the model of allergen-induced asthmatic reactions [97–99]. Roflumilast attenuates the late asthmatic reactions to allergens and allergen-induced airway hyperresponsiveness [99, 100]. It also inhibits allergen-induced airway neutrophilic inflammation which does not respond to treatment with corticosteroids [97, 101]. Moreover, a study has reported that a 4-week treatment with roflumilast of 500 mg once daily significantly inhibits exercise-induced asthma [102]. An oral PDE4 inhibitor, roflumilast, has an inhibitory effect on allergen-induced responses in patients with mild asthma and also reduces symptoms and lung function similar to a low dose of ICS [103]. To avoid the significant side effects which are big hurdle of the use of PDE4 inhibitor as a therapeutic agent for severe asthma, PDE4B-selective inhibitors or other delivery methods such as inhalation are under the development and clinical trials. Inhaled PDE3/4 inhibitors are also in development and might have the advantage of bronchodilatation through PDE3 inhibition [93, 104, 105].

6.2.4 ER Stress Modulator

The ER is the major site in cells, which is responsible for the synthesis, maturation, and trafficking of a wide range of proteins. When ER is stressed by some conditions such as increased demands in protein-folding load in ER lumen, cells evolve an adaptive response called unfolded protein response (UPR). However, when ER's adaptive responses failed to restore the capacity of ER to the normal physiologic status, ER has overloading state with abnormal functions which leads to ER stress [106, 107]. The ER stress is associated with pathogenic inflammatory mechanisms, in particular several diseases such as neurodegenerative disorders, metabolic disorders, cardiovascular diseases, malignancies, and respiratory disorders [64, 108–110]. Moreover, prolonged ER stress and UPR are implicated in chronic lung diseases, including cystic fibrosis, $\alpha 1$-antitrypsin deficiency, idiopathic pulmonary fibrosis, pulmonary hypertension, COPD, and bronchial asthma [111, 112]. As for severe asthma, recent interesting studies have been released in which ER stress and UPR inhibitor or chemical chaperone, 4-phenylbutyrate (4-PBA), substantially attenuated the steroid-resistant neutrophilic and eosinophilic asthmatic features in mice [64, 73]. Chemical chaperones, such as 4-PBA or tauroursodeoxycholic acid, were found to be extremely safe in preclinical studies and are now in clinical trials for various diseases [113–119]. These findings are very encouraging to pursue the clinical development of chemical chaperone as a therapeutic agent for patient with severe asthma, although so far, there are no studies for severe asthma to enter clinical trials. Furthermore, a recent study has introduced the possibility of inhaled chemical chaperone as treatment for allergic airway disease, suggesting its therapeutic potential with lower systemic toxicity for patients with severe asthma [120].

6.3 Endotype-Based Therapeutic Strategies

6.3.1 Type 2 Related Inflammation-Targeting Therapies

6.3.1.1 Anti-IgE Approach
Omalizumab, an anti-IgE monoclonal antibody (mAb), is the first targeted biologic therapeutic

approved for the treatment of moderate-to-severe persistent allergic asthma that remains uncontrolled despite high-dose inhaled corticosteroids plus other controller medications. Allergic asthma is believed to result from polarization of naive airway T cells to a Th2 phenotype, in which activated B cells produce and secrete IgE. The mode of action of anti-IgE mAb, omalizumab, is the blockade for IgE to bind IgE-receptor (FcεRI) on the surfaces of antigen-presenting cells, mast cells, and basophils through attaching to the Fc portion of free IgE with potent affinity leading to inhibition of subsequent inflammatory cell activation [121–123]. In addition, omalizumab prevent allergen-induced inflammatory responses as well as long-term consequences of allergen exposure such as airway remodeling, inflammatory cell recruitment, and Th2-biased inflammation [121–131]. Numerous clinical trials have demonstrated the clinical efficacy of omalizumab in reducing maintenance doses of oral corticosteroids and ICSs and in reducing exacerbations in patients including children with severe asthma, although no clinically measurable biomarkers have been found to predict a good response to omalizumab therapy [40, 124, 132–134]. In clinical practice, the use of omalizumab for adults and adolescents 12 years of age and older with moderate-to-severe allergic asthma was approved by US FDA in 2003 and by European Medicines Agency (EMA) in 2005 [135, 136]. In addition, the pediatric indication for omalizumab in asthmatic patients (use in children aged >6 years) was approved by the EMA and FDA in 2009 and 2016, respectively [135–137]. With the expansion of approval for the use of omalizumab, several international asthma guidelines and position papers also recommend omalizumab as an add-on therapy for the treatment of severe, IgE-mediated allergic asthma in patients including children whose asthma symptoms are uncontrolled despite optimal pharmacologic management and appropriate allergen avoidance [35, 125, 138–140]. Although anti-IgE was developed for allergic asthma defined by the presence of atopy and increased IgE levels, it is not always effective in these cases. Moreover, omalizumab

is so expensive and associated with side effects related to multiple injections, the risk of anaphylaxis, and even warning on cardiovascular risk. Thus, the development of biomarker to predict and monitor the pharmacologic responses and more improved formulation of anti-IgE agents are needed. Currently, the other anti-IgE mAb under development is ligelizumab which is a humanized anti-IgE antibody with a 50-fold higher affinity for IgE than omalizumab and shows good pharmacologic effects including reduction of concentration of IgE in allergic patients with well-controlled asthma [141]. In the future, the studies regarding the identification of biomarker to predict the therapeutic response, the development of more potent anti-IgE agents, and the use of anti-IgE mAb to non-atopic severe asthma with local IgE production are required for the precision medical treatment of severe asthma.

6.3.1.2 Inhibition of Cytokines: Targeting IL-4/IL-13 and IL-5, TSLP

Both IL-4 and IL-13 bind to the heterodimeric combination of the α1 chain of IL-13 receptor (IL-13Rα) and the α chain of IL-4 receptor (IL-4Rα), which leads to the signaling of both IL-4 and IL-13 [142]. In brief, IL-4Rα is the common receptor subchain for both IL-4 and IL-13, which is present in both the type 1 (dimerized with γ chain linked to activation of T cells) and type 2 (dimerized with IL-13 Rα) receptors. IL-4 activates both type 1 and type 2 receptors, whereas IL-13 only activates type 2 receptors. Thus, while IL-13 and IL-4 can promote IgE switching in B cells, T cell activation, and mast cell recruitment, IL-13 alone cannot differentiate T cells [143–145]. Pitrakinra is a mutant form of human IL-4 that blocks the ability of human IL-4 or IL-13 to bind to IL-4Rα. In phase II trials, nebulized pitrakinra for patients with mild atopic asthma reduced the late asthmatic response 3.7-fold compared with placebo [146]. However, as for moderate-to-severe asthma, pitrakinra and AMG317 which is a humanized mAb to IL-4Rα showed no effects on asthma outcomes including exacerbation and symptom score [147, 148]. Another humanized mAb to IL-4Rα, dupilumab was used for the first study to target a type 2-high phenotype, enrolling moderate-to-severe asthma patients with blood eosinophilia or sputum eosinophilia. In this study, dupilumab reduced asthma exacerbations and improved asthma control and lung function compared with placebo, when LABA was discontinued and ICS dose reduced and stopped [149]. Recently, a phase IIb dose-ranging study of dupilumab has been reported showing favorable results irrespective of baseline eosinophil count in patients with uncontrolled severe asthma and good safety profile as an add-on therapy [150]. In 2017, the use of dupilumab for patients with atopic dermatitis is approved by US FDA, and based on favorable results from several clinical studies, the approval for severe asthma is also expected in the near future.

Anti-IL-13 mAbs are lebrikizumab, tralokinumab, and GSK679586 which have been evaluated for their efficacy on the moderate-to-severe asthma, especially in type 2-high phenotype asthmatics [151–153]. Interestingly, lebrikizumab showed modest efficacy on exacerbations in patients with type 2 asthma identified by increased levels of serum IgE and blood eosinophilia [151]. However, in the same study, when type 2-high asthma was divided by serum periostin levels into the "high" and "low" groups, patients with high periostin levels treated with lebrikizumab had a more marked improvement in lung function, whereas those with low levels had no improvement. However, a recent report regarding replicate phase III clinical trials (NCT01867125, NCT01868061) has also revealed that lebrikizumab did not consistently show significant reduction in asthma exacerbations in biomarker-high patients [154]. Meanwhile, in cases of tralokinumab and GSK679586, they showed no significant efficacy on asthma outcomes such as asthma control, pulmonary function, or exacerbations [152, 153, 155].

The most advanced therapeutic target for type 2 inflammation is IL-5, which is an attractive target because it is an obligate cytokine for eosinophil maturation and survival. IL-5 acts as the most potent eosinophilic cytokine via binding its receptor with its receptor (IL-5 receptor α [IL-5Rα]) on eosinophils and some basophils [156, 157]. Eosinophilic inflammation is present with or without atopy, as a type 2-mediated response can occur following allergic sensitization, with consequent release of IL-5 from Th2 cells, or in response to stimulation of airway epithelial cells and infection through activation of the type 2 innate lymphoid cells (ILC2) [158, 159]. The IL-5 neutralizing antibodies, mepolizumab and reslizumab, have started to be prescribed by physicians and recommended as a therapeutic option by international guidelines for patient with severe asthma showing high blood/sputum eosinophil counts worldwide since the license was achieved in the United States and Europe in 2015 [160]. In earlier studies, mepolizumab reduced sputum and blood eosinophil counts compared with placebo but had no effect on response after allergen challenge. In addition, in patients with moderately severe asthma determined by disease severity, mepolizumab showed no beneficial effects on symptom control or exacerbations [161, 162]. In later studies, when patients with type 2 phenotype severe asthma showing eosinophilic asthma was enrolled selectively, mepolizumab reduced exacerbation rate, improved the symptom control, showed steroid sparing effects, and modestly improved lung function independent of administration routes (i.e., intravenous and subcutaneous) and doses [163–167]. Reslizumab was similarly studied in patients with poorly controlled asthma taking high-dose ICSs and additional controllers with persistent sputum eosinophils or blood eosinophils. Like mepolizumab, intravenous reslizumab decreased both blood and sputum eosinophil counts with increases in forced expiratory volume in 1 second (FEV1) and asthma control questionnaire (ACQ) scores and significant reduction of exacerbation compared with placebo [168, 169]. Benralizumab is a recombinant humanized mAb directed against IL-5Rα. Unlike mepolizumab and reslizumab, benralizumab binds to IL-5Rα on eosinophils and induces rapid depletion of eosinophils by antibody-dependent cell-mediated cytotoxicity through natural killer cells [170]. Two signature phase III clinical studies (SIROCCO study and CALIMA study) have revealed that benralizumab reduced asthma exacerbation, improved lung function, and achieved less asthma symptom score significantly compared to placebo [171, 172]. These results support for the earlier phase IIb study showing that in eosinophilic asthma, mean FEV1 and ACQ-6 improved by the benralizumab treatment [173]. Unlike mepolizumab and reslizumab which showed no significant effects on non-eosinophilic asthmatics, benralizumab showed some pharmacologic effects on asthmatic features in non-eosinophilic asthma which can be explained by the expression of IL-5Rα on other cells such as basophils and mast cells [156, 174]. Additional interesting point is that effects of anti-IL-5 mAbs and anti-IL-5Rα mAb on lung function are different in patients with severe asthma. Although there are not yet a direct head-to-head comparison studies, small effects on lung function were observed in the phase III study for mepolizumab [166], whereas effects on these outcomes were more robustly observed following treatment with reslizumab [169] and benralizumab [173]. The reason for these observations is unclear. However, some bronchoscopic biopsy data showed that benralizumab reduces bronchial mucosal eosinophilia to a greater extent than does mepolizumab [164, 175]. Given that benralizumab can induce apoptosis of eosinophils unlike mepolizumab, improvements in lung function might be related to the magnitude of the reduction in the airway eosinophilia.

TSLP is an IL-7-related cytokine secreted by airway epithelial cells on allergen and other stimuli; it has been recently described innate "alarmin" capable of regulating type 2 responses through activation of dendritic cells to release chemokines that recruit and activate Th2 cells [176]. TSLP levels are reported to be increased in human asthmatic airways compared with those of healthy control subjects, particularly in those with severe asthma [177]. Tezepelumab (AMG157, MEDI9929) is a human anti-TSLP mAb that binds human TSLP preventing receptor interaction [178]. Tezepelumab (AMG157) reduced allergen-induced bronchoconstriction and indexes of airway inflammation before and after allergen challenge. Very recently, phase II study to evaluate the efficacy and safety of tezepelumab in patients with severe asthma has been completed and awaits the results [179]. In addition, another phase II study is ongoing to investigate the effects on airway hyperresponsiveness measured by mannitol provocation test in patients with asthma already on daily treatment with ICS. In this study, secondary outcome is to evaluate cellular phenotypes including mast cells [180]. Nowadays, type 2-targeted therapy for severe asthma has moved into a new era thanks to newly emerging biologics. However, considerable challenges are also derived from these new therapeutic modalities including their long-term efficacy and safety, their comparative efficacy, patient selection related to biomarkers, and, finally, their cost-effectiveness.

6.3.2 Blockade of Lipid Mediators

A cysteinyl leukotriene-receptor antagonist (LTRAs) is an only antagonist against lipid mediators currently used in asthma therapy; however, these medications, montelukast and zafirlukast, are much less effective than ICSs and have little place as add-on therapy in patients with severe asthma [181, 182]. Apart from cysteinyl leukotrienes, leukotriene B4 (LTB4) is a potent chemoattractant for neutrophils, mast cells, and T cells, and its expression levels are increased in patients with severe asthma [183]. In addition, two receptors for LTB4, BLT1, and BLT2 are identified, and the two receptors differ in their affinity and specificity for LTB4 and in their expression pattern. BLT1 is a high-affinity receptor specific for LTB4 and usually expressed in leukocytes, whereas BLT2 is a low-affinity receptor and ubiquitously expressed [184]. Recently, papers have revealed that BLT1- and/or BLT2-targeting strategy led to attenuation of airway inflammation and airway hyperresponsiveness in a murine model of asthma [185, 186]. Several studies are ongoing to test the effects of inhibition of BLT1 and BLT2 on asthmatic features of severe disease status. First 5-lipoxygenase (5-LO) inhibitor, zileuton, has been used for treatment of asthma, but due to adverse effects, its immediate release tablet was withdrawn in 2008 [187]. Several novel 5-LO and 5-LO-activating protein inhibitors are currently in clinical development [40, 188]. GSK2190915, a potent 5-lipoxygenase-activating protein inhibitor, prevents the synthesis of leukotrienes and 5-oxo-eicosatetraenoic acid (5-oxo-ETE). It attenuated the early and late asthmatic responses in mild asthmatic patients. In addition, there was a statistically significant attenuation of allergen-induced sputum eosinophil count. This study suggested the therapeutic potential of 5-LO-activating protein inhibitor for patients with asthma although further study is needed, in particular regarding the effects on severe asthma [189]. Prostaglandin D2, released form mast cells, Th2 cells, and dendritic cells during allergen-induced reactions, activates a chemoattractant receptor-homologous molecule expressed on Th2 cells (CRTh2), present on Th2 cells, ILC2s, and eosinophils, and induces the chemotaxis of these cells [190]. Production of Th2 cytokines by ILC2s is also stimulated by activation of CRTh2 receptor [191]. In addition, some evidence has shown that the expression of prostaglandin D2 was increased in patients with severe asthma [192]. Based on these backgrounds, several CRTH2 antagonists are now in clinical development for asthma, including AMG-853, OC000459, MK-7246, BI671800, and fevipiprant (QAW039) [193]. Considerable data on favorable outcome in asthmatic patients including eosinophilic phenotype has been gathered; however, there is still controversy on the effects of CRTh2 antagonists on severe asthmatic features to date [194–197]. In fact, while AMG 853 did not improve asthma symptoms or lung function in patients with uncontrolled moderate-to-severe asthma, BI671900 showed small effects on lung function in symptomatic patients, and a phase II study with fevipiprant has recently revealed its beneficial effects on lung function and eosinophilic inflammation in sputum and bronchial biopsied tissues. Not yet, the findings from phase III studies have been released.

6.3.3 Chemokine Receptor Antagonists: CCR3 and CCR4

Chemokines attract inflammatory cells such as mast cells, eosinophils, and TH2 cells into the airways, and they exert function through their receptors, chemokine receptors which are surface molecules that belong to the family of seven transmembrane domain receptors, designated G protein-coupled receptors (GPCRs) [198]. Among 18 family members of chemokine receptor, the major focus of interest in asthmatic patients has been the chemokine receptor CCR3, which is predominantly expressed on eosinophils and mediates the chemotactic response to CCL11 (eotaxin), which is secreted in asthma. Several small-molecule inhibitors of CCR3 have been in clinical development, but their effects in asthmatic patients have not yet been reported because they have usually been discontinued because of toxicology problems. An inhaled antisense oligonucleotide that targets CCR3 has some effect in reducing sputum eosinophils, but results are difficult to interpret because IL-5 and GM-CSF β chain antisense were co-administered [199]. In terms of other chemokine receptors, the CCR2, CCR4, CCR5, CCR6, CCR8, and CXCR4 have been implicated in asthma, especially type 2-related responses. Substantial experimental data support the potential of chemokine receptor antagonists as therapeutic agent for asthma, but controversy still remained, and there are no definitive results from clinical trials [200]. A defucosylated antibody to CCR4 (mogamulizumab) results in prolonged cytotoxic effects on Th2 cells, marked and prolonged depletion of Th2 cells, and reduced lung inflammation in animal models. This antibody was granted approval for the treatment of relapsed or refractory adult T cell lymphoma in 2012 and is now in early clinical trials for asthma [201, 202]. In addition, another small-molecule antagonist, an indazole arylsulfonamide GSK2239633, appears to have progressed to clinical trials [203].

6.4 Non-type 2-Related Inflammation-Targeting Therapies

6.4.1 Anti-tumor Necrosis Factor α (TNF-α)

TNF-α is a pro-inflammatory cytokine leading to non-type 2 neutrophilic inflammation. Blockade of TNF-α is highly effective in patients with the type 1-associated chronic inflammatory disease such as rheumatoid arthritis. In murine models inhalation of TNF-α contributes to neutrophilic inflammation and bronchial hyperresponsiveness [204]. Etanercept is a soluble recombinant dimer protein consisting of two human TNF-α receptors fused with the Fc domain of human IgG1 and showed clinical improvements in airway hyperresponsiveness measured by methacholine provocation test, quality of life scores, and lung function, ACQ scores, and reduction of the use of rescue medication in patients with steroid-refractory asthma [205, 206]. Infliximab is an anti-TNF-α mAb which was also studied in patients with non-phenotyped asthma. In patients with moderate asthma, infliximab treatment was associated with a decrease in diurnal peak expiratory flow variation and decreased asthma exacerbations [207]. However, in a large-scale study in adults with uncontrolled severe persistent asthma using golimumab, the anti-TNF-α humanized mAb had no overall beneficial effects [208]. On the contrary, serious side effects associated with golimumab were reported including an increased frequency of infections and malignancies compared with placebo resulting in premature termination of this clinical trial. Therefore, current evidence suggests that the risk of anti-TNF-α therapies outweighs benefit in severe asthma.

6.4.2 Anti-interleukins: IL-17

IL-17A is one of the key players in neutrophilic airway inflammation using animal models of asthma induced by various allergen and stimuli [67, 209]. Additionally, a murine model of steroid-resistant neutrophilic asthma showed significant increases of IL-17A and murine IL-8 (CXCL8) homolog KC in lung tissues [64]. Indeed, elevated levels of IL-17A were found in the sputum and in BAL of patients with asthma, and many studies have confirmed these findings and demonstrated a positive correlation between IL-17A production and asthma severity [210–214].

Brodalumab is a human anti-IL-17RA monoclonal antibody which blocks receptor binding of IL-17A and IL-17F but also blocks binding of the type 2-associated cytokine IL-17E/IL-25 [214]. Against many expectations, despite good results in preclinical studies, brodalumab had no effect on asthma control scores, symptom-free days, and FEV1 in non-phenotyped patients with inadequately controlled moderate-to-severe asthma who were receiving inhaled corticosteroid therapy. Although a phenotyped subgroup showing a high bronchial reversibility exhibited a significant improvement in ACQ score, the results had uncertain significance [215]. Thus, a follow-up phase IIb study focusing on this phenotype had been performed, but it was stopped because of a lack of reported efficacy in an interim analysis. There has been no further development of this antibody in asthma. Secukinumab (AIN457), an anti-IL-17 mAb that selectively neutralizes IL-17A, has been tested in phase II trials in asthmatic subjects who are not adequately controlled with ICSs and long-acting b2-agonists (NCT01478360). This study also has been terminated with no significant beneficial effects on patient group. Currently, it is hypothesized that these disappointing clinical results can be derived from the absence of selection based on an IL-17- or neutrophil-related criterion leading to the inclusion of many patients with Th2 high severe asthma in these trials who are less likely to respond to an IL-17-targeted therapy.

6.4.3 Inflammasome Inhibitor

NLRP3 inflammasome activation is critical for the induction of allergic airway inflammation in bronchial asthma [216, 217], with increased understanding of how adaptive and innate immunity generates downstream pathology of allergic inflammation [218]. Furthermore, recent interesting studies have revealed that steroid-resistant neutrophilic asthmatic manifestations were significantly controlled by the NLRP3 inflammasome activation, and the severe asthmatic symptoms were dramatically attenuated by the blockade of IL-1β or inflammasome inhibitor, MCC950. Moreover, that increased NLRP3 and IL-1β sputum gene expression was strongly associated with increasing asthma severity in humans, suggesting that the NLRP3 inflammasome is important in human disease as well [63, 219]. In fact, based on transcriptomic analysis with sputum from patients with moderate-to-severe asthma, non-Th2 phenotypes of severe asthma included two transcriptome-associated clusters (TACs); one cluster is characterized by IFN-γ, TNF-α, and inflammasome-associated genes, and the other cluster is represented by genes of metabolic pathways, ubiquitination, and mitochondrial function [220]. To date, there is no interventional clinical data regarding targeting NLRP3 inflammasome in steroid-refractory severe asthma; however, it can be a very promising target for the control of severe asthma, especially non-eosinophilic type.

6.4.4 Chemokine Receptor Antagonists: CXCR2

CXCL8 is a chemokine involved in the chemoattraction and activation of neutrophils through the CXCR2 receptor. An oral CXCR1/CXCR2 antagonist, navarixin (SCH-527123), is effective in blocking ozone-induced sputum neutrophilia in healthy subjects, and it also reduced sputum neutrophilia in adults with severe asthma, with a modest reduction in mild exacerbations, but did not improve asthma control [221, 222]. In addition, several CXCR2 receptor-targeting agents such as reparixin, AZD8309, SB656933, GSK1325756, and AZD5069 have developed and entered to clinical trials for various inflammatory disorders including infectious airway inflammation [223].

6.5 Clinical Comorbidities-Based Therapeutic Modalities

6.5.1 Antifungal Agents: Allergic Bronchopulmonary Aspergillosis (ABPA) and Severe Asthma with Fungal Sensitization (SAFS)

SAFS and ABPA encompass two closely related subgroups of patients with severe allergic asthma. Pulmonary disease is due to pronounced host inflammatory responses to noninvasive subclinical endobronchial infection with filamentous fungi, usually *Aspergillus fumigatus* [224]. The use of antifungal agents including oral triazoles and inhaled amphotericin B has been evaluated for the possibility as an add-on therapeutic modality in patient with ABPA or SAFS. First, several clinical trials suggest an anti-inflammatory benefit of itraconazole in ABPA in asthma patients, which may be due to a reduction in fungal burden or perhaps other non-antimicrobial mechanisms [225–230]. Moreover, the use of azoles for ABPA in asthma patients was recommended by the Cochrane collaboration [231, 232]. As for patients with SAFS, the effects of azoles have recently been tested clinically. The therapeutic effects included improvement of asthma symptom score and lung function and reduction of serum IgE levels [233]. Additionally, similar success in treating SAFS in children with itraconazole has also been reported [234, 235]. In addition, nebulized or inhaled formulations of liposomal amphotericin B can be tried in order to reduce the risks of side effects including medication interactions. This is quite promising in the field if the risk does not outweigh the benefits. However, to date, the clinical results regarding the use of amphotericin B for patients with ABPA or SAFS are so limited. Two recent reports have released about the nebulized use of amphotericin or liposomal amphotericin in patient with ABPA and cystic fibrosis resulting in favorable outcomes [236, 237], while there have been no published reports of inhaled amphotericin use in SAFS.

6.5.2 Macrolides: Infections and Bronchiectasis

Studies have reported that some patients with severe asthma are chronically infected with atypical bacteria, such as *Mycoplasma pneumoniae* and *Chlamydia pneumoniae* [238]. However, the long-term treatment of macrolide, clarithromycin, did not show any significant improvement of asthma control, and the clinical results regarding this issue remained to be controversial [239, 240]. In terms of severe asthma combined with pulmonary structural disorders, it is very worthy to note that maintenance treatment with low-dose macrolides has been shown to reduce neutrophilic inflammation in the airways of patients suffering from various chronic diseases, mainly cystic fibrosis (CF) and non-CF bronchiectasis [241]. In a randomized double-blind placebo-controlled trial, the treatment with low-dose azithromycin resulted in the significant reduction of exacerbation rate but not lower respiratory infections in the neutrophilic subgroup of asthmatic patients [242]. To conclude the role of macrolide in severe asthma, more prospective trials are needed.

6.5.3 Intranasal Spray and Intranasal Inhalation of Corticosteroids: Allergic Rhinitis (AR)

To date, there is limited information on the additional effects of intranasal corticosteroid treatment as add-on modalities on asthma outcome of patients with severe asthma. A meta-analysis reported that intranasal corticosteroid medications significantly improve some asthma-specific outcome measures in patients suffering from both AR and asthma. However, there were no significant changes in asthma outcomes with the addition of intranasal corticosteroid spray to orally inhaled corticosteroids. The therapeutic effect was most pronounced with intranasal corticosteroid sprays when patients were not on daily orally inhaled corticosteroids or when corticosteroid medications were inhaled through the nose into the lungs [243]. Prospective research is needed for the effective management of severe asthma with AR through the selection of adequate inhaled technique or the dual inhaled therapy.

6.5.4 IFN-β: Viral Infection-Associated Asthma Exacerbation

Exacerbations of asthma are most commonly caused by respiratory viruses [244, 245] and are responsible for emergency department visits and considerable fatalities, especially in more severe disease [246–248]. Among various viruses, rhinoviruses are by far the most common cause of exacerbation. A great deal of research has hypothesized that this increased asthma susceptibility is related to an impaired interferon (IFN) response to infection [249]. In fact, a previous study has revealed that when infected with rhinoviruses, the asthmatic bronchial epithelium failed to mount an effective innate immune response involving IFN-β [250]. Intranasal administration of SNG001, recombinant IFN-β1a formulated as an aqueous solution starting with symptom onset, failed to significantly decrease the severity of exacerbation. However, analysis of the moderate-to-severe people with asthma suggested a beneficial clinical effect of treatment presented as reduction in ACQ-6 score in patients treated with IFN-β [251]. A further powered phase II clinical trial focusing on more severe asthma patients has been recently completed and waits for the results (NCT02491684).

Figure 6.1 summarizes the content of this chapter.

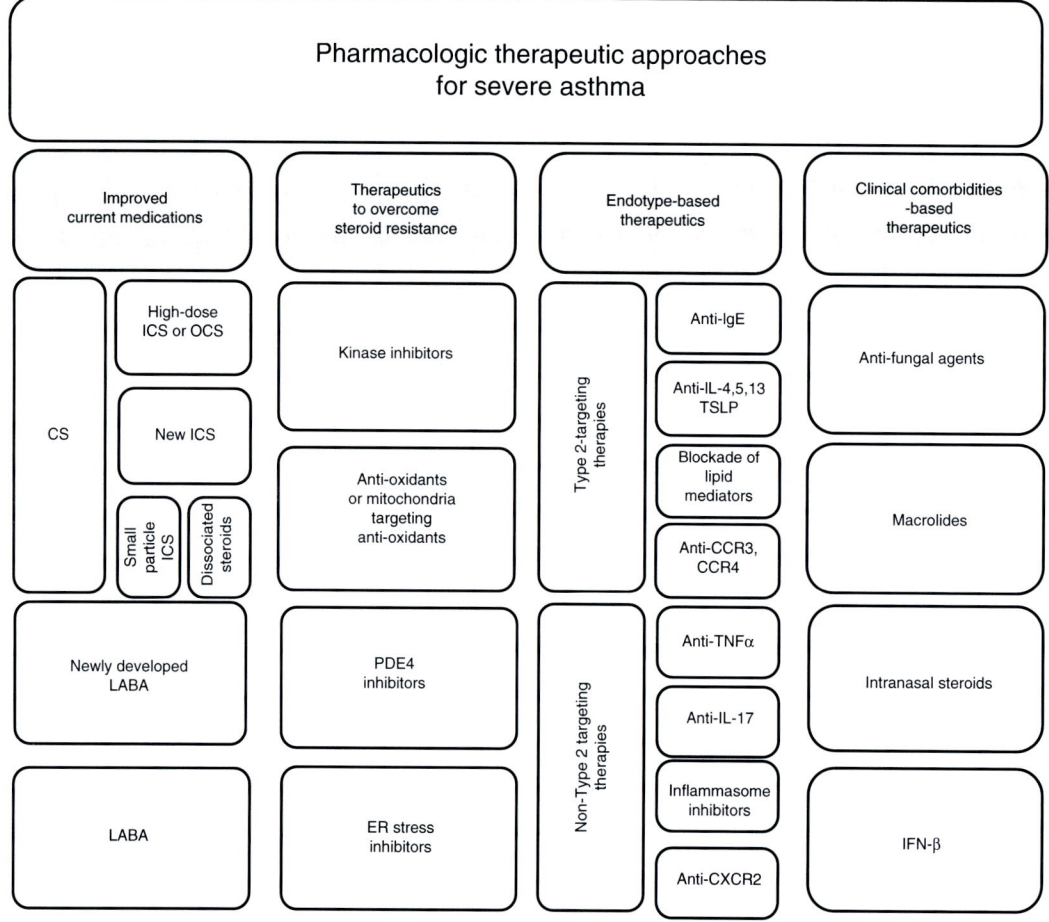

Fig. 6.1 Summary of pharmacologic therapeutics for severe asthma

References

1. Global Initiative for Asthma (GINA). Global strategy for asthma management and prevention (updated 2017). 2017. http://www.ginasthma.org. Accessed 5 May 2017.
2. Adams NP, Bestall JC, Jones P, Lasserson TJ, Griffiths B, Cates CJ, et al. Fluticasone at different doses for chronic asthma in adults and children. Cochrane Database Syst Rev. 2008;4:CD003534.
3. Bateman ED, Boushey HA, Bousquet J, Busse WW, Clark TJ, Pauwels RA, et al. Can guideline-defined asthma control be achieved? The Gaining Optimal Asthma Control study. Am J Respir Crit Care Med. 2004;170(8):836–44.
4. Cates CJ, Lasserson TJ. Combination formoterol and budesonide as maintenance and reliever therapy versus inhaled steroid maintenance for chronic asthma in adults and children. Cochrane Database Syst Rev. 2009;2:CD007313.
5. Dweik RA, Boggs PB, Erzurum SC, Irvin CG, Leigh MW, Lundberg JO, et al. An official ATS clinical practice guideline: interpretation of exhaled nitric oxide levels (FENO) for clinical applications. Am J Respir Crit Care Med. 2011;184(5):602–15.
6. Nave R. Clinical pharmacokinetic and pharmacodynamic profile of inhaled ciclesonide. Clin Pharmacokinet. 2009;48(4):243–52.
7. Gentile DA, Skoner DP. New asthma drugs: small molecule inhaled corticosteroids. Curr Opin Pharmacol. 2010;10(3):260–5.
8. Contoli M, Bousquet J, Fabbri LM, Magnussen H, Rabe KF, Siafakas NM, et al. The small airways and distal lung compartment in asthma and COPD: a time for reappraisal. Allergy. 2010;65(2):141–51.
9. Hodgson D, Anderson J, Reynolds C, Meakin G, Bailey H, Pavord I, et al. A randomised controlled trial of small particle inhaled steroids in refractory eosinophilic asthma (SPIRA). Thorax. 2015;70(6):559–65.

10. Biggadike K. Fluticasone furoate/fluticasone propionate—different drugs with different properties. Clin Respir J. 2011;5(3):183–4.

11. Allen A, Pierre LN, Rousell VM. Fluticasone furoate (FF) a novel inhaled corticosteroid demonstrates prolonged lung absorption kinetics in man. Am J Respir Crit Care Med. 2010;181:A5408.

12. van den Berge M, Luijk B, Bareille P, Dallow N, Postma DS, Lammers JW, et al. Prolonged protection of the new inhaled corticosteroid fluticasone furoate against AMP hyperresponsiveness in patients with asthma. Allergy. 2010;65(12):1531–5.

13. Keith PK, Scadding GK. Are intranasal corticosteroids all equally consistent in managing ocular symptoms of seasonal allergic rhinitis? Curr Med Res Opin. 2009;25(8):2021–41.

14. Gueron B, Demoly P, Piercy J, Small M. Do patients on intranasal fluticasone furoate, mometasone furoate and fluticasone propionate experience similar numbers of symptom-free days and quality of life? A cross-sectional study in three European countries. Allergy 2010;65 (Suppl 92):156.

15. Okobu K, Nakashima M, Miyake N, Komatsubara M, Okuda M. Comparison of fluticasone furoate and fluticasone propionate for the treatment of Japanese cedar pollinosis. Allergy Asthma Proc. 2009;30(1):84–94.

16. Woodcock A, Bleecker ER, Lötvall J, O'Byrne PM, Bateman ED, Medley H, et al. Efficacy and safety of fluticasone furoate/vilanterol compared with fluticasone propionate/salmeterol combination in adult and adolescent patients with persistent asthma. Chest. 2013;144(4):1222–9.

17. Schacke H, Berger M, Rehwinkel H, Asadullah K. Selective glucocorticoid receptor agonists (SEGRAs): novel ligands with an improved therapeutic index. Mol Cell Endocrinol. 2007;275(1–2):109–17.

18. De Bosscher K. Selective glucocorticoid receptor modulators. J Steroid Biochem Mol Biol. 2010;120(2–3):96–104.

19. Cazzola M, Coppola A, Rogliani P, Matera MG. Novel glucocorticoid receptor agonists in the treatment of asthma. Expert Opin Investig Drugs. 2015;24(11):1473–82.

20. Rossi A, van der Molen T, del Olmo R, Papi A, Wehbe L, Quinn M, del Olmo R, et al. INSTEAD: a randomised switch trial of indacaterol versus salmeterol/fluticasone in moderate COPD. Eur Respir J. 2014;44(6):1548–56.

21. Ferguson GT, Feldman GJ, Hofbauer P, Hamilton A, Allen L, Korducki L, et al. Efficacy and safety of olodaterol once daily delivered via Respimat® in patients with GOLD 2–4 COPD: results from two replicate 48-week studies. Int J Chron Obstruct Pulmon Dis. 2014;9:629–45.

22. Chapman KR, Rennard SI, Dogra A, Owen R, Lassen C, Kramer B, et al. Long-term safety and efficacy of indacaterol, a long-acting β_2-agonist, in subjects with COPD: a randomized, placebo-controlled study. Chest. 2011;140(1):68–75.

23. Hanania NA, Feldman G, Zachgo W, Shim JJ, Crim C, Sanford L, et al. The efficacy and safety of the novel long-acting β2 agonist vilanterol in patients with COPD: a randomized placebo-controlled trial. Chest. 2012;142(1):119–27.

24. Beasley RW, Donohue JF, Mehta R, Nelson HS, Clay M, Moton A, et al. Effect of once-daily indacaterol maleate/mometasone furoate on exacerbation risk in adolescent and adult asthma: a double-blind randomised controlled trial. BMJ Open. 2015;5(2):e006131.

25. Raemdonck K, de Alba J, Birrell MA, Grace M, Maher SA, Irvin CG, et al. A role for sensory nerves in the late asthmatic response. Thorax. 2012;67(1):19–25.

26. Kummer W, Lips KS, Pfeil U. The epithelial cholinergic system of the airways. Histochem Cell Biol. 2008,130(2):219–34.

27. Bateman ED, Rennard S, Barnes PJ, Dicpinigaitis PV, Gosens R, Gross NJ, et al. Alternative mechanisms for tiotropium. Pulm Pharmacol Ther. 2009;22(6):533–42.

28. Ohta S, Oda N, Yokoe T, Tanaka A, Yamamoto Y, Watanabe Y, et al. Effect of tiotropium bromide on airway inflammation and remodelling in a mouse model of asthma. Clin Exp Allergy. 2010;40(8):1266–75.

29. Bos IS, Gosens R, Zuidhof AB, Schaafsma D, Halayko AJ, Meurs H, et al. Inhibition of allergen-induced airway remodelling by tiotropium and budesonide: a comparison. Eur Respir J. 2007;30(4):653–61.

30. Park HW, Yang MS, Park CS, Kim TB, Moon HB, Min KU, et al. Additive role of tiotropium in severe asthmatics and Arg16Gly in ADRB2 as a potential marker to predict response. Allergy. 2009;64(5):778–83.

31. Kerstjens HA, Disse B, Schroder-Babo W, Bantje TA, Gahlemann M, Sigmund R, et al. Tiotropium improves lung function in patients with severe uncontrolled asthma: a randomized controlled trial. J Allergy Clin Immunol. 2011;128(2):308–14.

32. Peters SP, Kunselman SJ, Icitovic N, Moore WC, Pascual R, Ameredes BT, et al. Tiotropium bromide step-up therapy for adults with uncontrolled asthma. N Engl J Med. 2010;363(18):1715–26.

33. Bateman ED, Kornmann O, Schmidt P, Pivovarova A, Engel M, Fabbri LM, et al. Tiotropium is non-inferior to salmeterol in maintaining improved lung function in B16-Arg/Arg patients with asthma. J Allergy Clin Immunol. 2011;128(2):315–22.

34. Kerstjens HAM, Engel M, Dahl R, Paggiaro P, Beck E, Vandewalker M, et al. Tiotropium in asthma poorly controlled with standard combination therapy. N Engl J Med. 2012;367(13):1198–207.

35. Global Initiative for Asthma (GINA). Global strategy for asthma management and prevention (updated 2016). 2016. http://www.ginasthma.org. Accessed 5 May 2017.

36. Hansel TT, Neighbour H, Erin EM, Tan AJ, Tennant RC, Maus JG, et al. Glycopyrrolate causes prolonged bronchoprotection and bronchodilatation in patients with asthma. Chest. 2005;128(4):1974–9.

37. Lee LA, Briggs A, Edwards LD, Yang S, Pascoe S. A randomized, three-period crossover study of umeclidinium as monotherapy in adult patients with asthma. Respir Med. 2015;109(1):63–73.

38. Lee LA, Yang S, Kerwin E, Trivedi R, Edwards LD, Pascoe S, et al. The effect of fluticasone furoate/umeclidinium in adult patients with asthma: a randomized, dose-ranging study. Respir Med. 2015;109(1):54–62.

39. Adcock IM, Chung KF, Caramori G, Ito L. Kinase inhibitors and airway inflammation. Eur J Pharmacol. 2006;533(1–3):118–32.

40. Barnes PJ. Severe asthma: advances in current management and future therapy. J Allergy Clin Immunol. 2012;129(1):48–59.

41. Mercado N, Hakim A, Kobayashi Y, Meah S, Usmani OS, Chung KF, et al. Restoration of corticosteroid sensitivity by p38 mitogen activated protein kinase inhibition in peripheral blood mononuclear cells from severe asthma. PLoS One. 2012;7(7):e41582.

42. Ismaili N, Garabedian MJ. Modulation of glucocorticoid receptor function via phosphorylation. Ann N Y Acad Sci. 2004;1024:86–101.

43. Loke TK, Mallett KH, Ratoff J, O'Connor BJ, Ying S, Meng Q, et al. Systemic glucocorticoid reduces bronchial mucosal activation of activator protein 1 components in glucocorticoid-sensitive but not glucocorticoid-resistant asthmatic patients. J Allergy Clin Immunol. 2006;118(2):368–75.

44. Goleva E, Kisich KO, Leung DY. A role for STAT5 in the pathogenesis of IL-2-induced glucocorticoid resistance. J Immunol. 2002;169(10):5934–40.

45. To Y, Ito K, Kizawa Y, Failla M, Ito M, Kusama T, et al. Targeting phosphoinositide-3-kinase-d with theophylline reverses corticosteroid insensitivity in COPD. Am J Respir Crit Care Med. 2010;182(7):897–904.

46. Bhavsar P, Hew M, Khorasani N, Alfonso T, Barnes PJ, Adcock I, et al. Relative corticosteroid insensitivity of alveolar macrophages in severe asthma compared to non-severe asthma. Thorax. 2008;63(9):784–90.

47. Barnes PJ, Adcock IM. Glucocorticoid resistance in inflammatory diseases. Lancet. 2009;373(9678):1905–17.

48. Sher ER, Leung DY, Surs W, Kam JC, Zieg G, Kamada AK, et al. Steroid-resistant asthma. Cellular mechanisms contributing to inadequate response to glucocorticoid therapy. J Clin Invest. 1994;93(1):33–9.

49. Irusen E, Matthews JG, Takahashi A, Barnes PJ, Chung KF, Adcock IM, et al. p38 mitogen-activated protein kinase-induced glucocorticoid receptor phosphorylation reduces its activity: role in steroid-insensitive asthma. J Allergy Clin Immunol. 2002;109(4):649–57.

50. Cuenda A, Rousseau S. p38 MAP-kinases pathway regulation, function and role in human diseases. Biochim Biophys Acta. 2007;1773(8):1358–75.

51. Hammaker D, Firestein GS. "Go upstream, young man": lessons learned from the p38 saga. Ann Rheum Dis. 2010;69(Suppl 1):i77–82.

52. Duan W, Chan JH, McKay K, Crosby JR, Choo HH, Leung BP, et al. Inhaled p38alpha mitogen-activated protein kinase antisense oligonucleotide attenuates asthma in mice. Am J Respir Crit Care Med. 2005;171(6):571–8.

53. Millan DS, Bunnage ME, Burrows JL, Butcher KJ, Dodd PG, Evans TJ, et al. Design and synthesis of inhaled p38 inhibitors for the treatment of chronic obstructive pulmonary disease. J Med Chem. 2011;54(22):7797–814.

54. Kim SR, Lee KS, Park SJ, Min KH, Lee MH, Lee KA, et al. A novel dithiol amide CB3 attenuates allergic airway disease through negative regulation of p38 mitogen-activated protein kinase. Am J Respir Crit Care Med. 2011;183(8):1015–524.

55. Barnes PJ. Therapeutic approaches to asthma–chronic obstructive pulmonary disease overlap syndromes. J Allergy Clin Immunol. 2015;136(3):531–45.

56. Hart LA, Krishnan VL, Adcock IM, Barnes PJ, Chung KF. Activation and localization of transcription factor, nuclear factor-kB, in asthma. Am J Respir Crit Care Med. 1998;158(5 Pt 1):1585–92.

57. Caramori G, Romagnoli M, Casolari P, Bellettato C, Casoni G, Boschetto P, et al. Nuclear localisation of p65 in sputum macrophages but not in sputum neutrophils during COPD exacerbations. Thorax. 2003;58(4):348–51.

58. Lee YC, Lee KS, Park SJ, Park HS, Lim JS, Park KH, et al. Blockade of airway hyperresponsiveness and inflammation in a murine model of asthma by a prodrug of cysteine, L-2-oxothiazolidine-4-carboxylic acid. FASEB J. 2004;18(15):1917–9.

59. Lee KS, Kim SR, Park SJ, Park HS, Min KH, Jin SM, et al. Peroxisome proliferator activated receptor-gamma modulates reactive oxygen species generation and activation of nuclear factor-kappaB and hypoxia-inducible factor 1alpha in allergic airway disease of mice. Allergy Clin Immunol. 2006;118(1):120–7.

60. Lee KS, Kim SR, Park SJ, Min KH, Lee KY, Jin SM, et al. Antioxidant down-regulates interleukin-18 expression in asthma. Mol Pharmacol. 2006;70(4):1184–93.

61. Lee KS, Kim SR, Park HS, Park SJ, Min KH, Lee KY, et al. A novel thiol compound, N-acetylcysteine amide, attenuates allergic airway disease by regulating activation of NF-kappaB and hypoxia-inducible factor-1alpha. Exp Mol Med. 2007;39(6):756–68.

62. Park SJ, Lee KS, Lee SJ, Kim SR, Park SY, Jeon MS, et al. L-2-Oxothiazolidine-4-carboxylic acid or α-lipoic acid attenuates airway remodeling: involvement of nuclear factor-κB (NF-κB), nuclear factor erythroid 2p45-related factor-2 (Nrf2), and

hypoxia-inducible factor (HIF). Int J Mol Sci. 2012;13(7):7915–37.

63. Kim SR, Kim DI, Kim SH, Lee H, Lee KS, Cho SH, et al. NLRP3 inflammasome activation by mitochondrial ROS in bronchial epithelial cells is required for allergic inflammation. Cell Death Dis. 2014;5:e1498.

64. Kim SR, Kim DI, Kang MR, Lee KS, Park SY, Jeong JS, et al. Endoplasmic reticulum stress influences bronchial asthma pathogenesis by modulating nuclear factor κB activation. J Allergy Clin Immunol. 2013;132(6):1397–408.

65. Kwak YG, Song CH, Yi HK, Hwang PH, Kim JS, Lee KS, et al. Involvement of PTEN in airway hyperresponsiveness and inflammation in bronchial asthma. J Clin Invest. 2003;111(7):1083–92.

66. Lee KS, Park SJ, Kim SR, Min KH, Jin SM, Puri KD, et al. Phosphoinositide 3-kinase-delta inhibitor reduces vascular permeability in a murine model of asthma. J Allergy Clin Immunol. 2006;118(2):403–9.

67. Kim SR, Lee KS, Park SJ, Min KH, Lee KY, Choe YH, et al. PTEN down-regulates IL-17 expression in a murine model of toluene diisocyanate-induced airway disease. J Immunol. 2007;179(10):6820–9.

68. Lee KS, Park SJ, Kim SR, Min KH, Lee KY, Choe YH, et al. Inhibition of VEGF blocks TGF-beta1 production through a PI3K/Akt signalling pathway. Eur Respir J. 2008;31(3):523–31.

69. Lee KS, Kim SR, Park SJ, Min KH, Lee KY, Choe YH, et al. Mast cells can mediate vascular permeability through regulation of the PI3K-HIF-1alpha-VEGF axis. Am J Respir Crit Care Med. 2008;178(8):787–97.

70. Park SJ, Min KH, Lee YC. Phosphoinositide 3-kinase delta inhibitor as a novel therapeutic agent in asthma. Respirology. 2008;13(6):764–71.

71. Kim SR, Lee KS, Park HS, Park SJ, Min KH, Moon H, et al. HIF-1α inhibition ameliorates an allergic airway disease via VEGF suppression in bronchial epithelium. Eur J Immunol. 2010;40(10):2858–69.

72. Kim DI, Kim SR, Kim HJ, Lee SJ, Lee HB, Park SJ, et al. PI3K-γ inhibition ameliorates acute lung injury through regulation of IκBα/NF κB pathway and innate immune responses. J Clin Immunol. 2012;32(2):340–51.

73. Lee KS, Jeong JS, Kim SR, Cho SH, Kolliputi N, Ko YH, et al. Phosphoinositide 3-kinase-δ regulates fungus-induced allergic lung inflammation through endoplasmic reticulum stress. Thorax. 2016;71(1):52–63.

74. Horak F, Puri KD, Steiner BH, Holes L, Xing G, Zieglmayer P, et al. Randomized phase 1 study of the phosphatidylinositol 3-kinase δ inhibitor idelalisib in patients with allergic rhinitis. J Allergy Clin Immunol. 2016;137(6):1733–41.

75. Nohl H, Kozlov AV, Gille L, Staniek K. Cell respiration and formation of reactive oxygen species: facts and artefacts. Biochem Soc Trans. 2003;31(Pt 6):1308–11.

76. Liu PL, Chen YL, Chen YH, Lin SJ, Kou YR. Wood smoke extract induces oxidative stress-mediated caspase-independent apoptosis in human lung endothelial cells: role of AIF and EndoG. Am J Physiol Lung Cell Mol Physiol. 2005;289(5):L739–49.

77. Vayssier-Taussat M, Camilli T, Aron Y, Meplan C, Hainaut P, Polla BS, et al. Effects of tobacco smoke and benzo[a]pyrene on human endothelial cell and monocyte stress responses. Am J Physiol Heart Circ Physiol. 2001;280(3):H1293–300.

78. Wilson MR, Lightbody JH, Donaldson K, Sales J, Stone V. Interactions between ultrafine particles and transition metals in vivo and in vitro. Toxicol Appl Pharmacol. 2002;184(3):172–9.

79. Park HS, Kim SR, Kim JO, Lee YC. The roles of phytochemicals in bronchial asthma. Molecules. 2010;15(10):6810–34.

80. Barnes PJ. Reactive oxygen species in asthma. Eur Respir Rev. 2000;10:240–3.

81. Lee KS, Kim SR, Park SJ, Park HS, Min KH, Lee MH, et al. Hydrogen peroxide induces vascular permeability via regulation of vascular endothelial growth factor. Am J Respir Cell Mol Biol. 2006;35(2):190–7.

82. Cho YJ, Seo MS, Kim JK, Lim Y, Chae G, Ha KS, et al. Silica-induced generation of reactive oxygen species in Rat2 fibroblasts: role in activation of mitogen-activated protein kinase. Biochem Biophys Res Commun. 1999;262(3):708–12.

83. Ding M, Shi X, Dong Z, Chen F, Lu Y, Castranova V, et al. Freshly fractured crystalline silica induces activator protein-1 activation through ERKs and p38 MAPK. J Biol Chem. 1999;274(43):30611–6.

84. Lopez-Ilasaca M, Crespo P, Pellici PG, Gutkind JS, Wetzker R. Linkage of G protein coupled receptors to the MAPK signaling pathway through PI 3-kinase gamma. Science. 1997;275(5298):394–7.

85. Lee KS, Park HS, Park SJ, Kim SR, Min KH, Jin SM, et al. An antioxidant modulates expression of receptor activator of NF-κB in asthma. Exp Mol Med. 2006;38(3):217–29.

86. Schenk H, Klein M, Erdbrügger W, Dröge W, Schulze-Osthoff K. Distinct effects of thioredoxin and antioxidants on the activation of transcription factors NF-κB and AP-1. Proc Natl Acad Sci U S A. 1994;91(5):1672–6.

87. Harper R, Wu K, Chang MM, Yoneda K, Pan R, Reddy SP, et al. Activation of nuclear factor-kappa b transcriptional activity in airway epithelial cells by thioredoxin but not by Nacetyl-cysteine and glutathione. Am J Respir Cell Mol Biol. 2001;25(2):178–85.

88. Shaulian E, Karin M. AP-1 as a regulator of cell life and death. Nat Cell Biol. 2002;4(5):E131–6.

89. Tikoo K, Lau SS, Monks TJ. Histone H2 phosphorylation is coupled to poly(ADPribosylation) during reactive oxygen species-induced cell death in renal proximal tubular epithelial cells. Mol Pharmacol. 2001;60(2):394–402.

90. Zor U, Ferber E, Gergely P, Szücs K, Dombrádi V, Goldman R, et al. Reactive oxygen species mediate phorbol ester-regulated tyrosine phosphorylation and phospholipase A2 activation: potentiation by vanadate. Biochem J. 1993;295(Pt 3):879–88.

91. Goldman R, Ferber E, Zort U. Reactive oxygen species are involved in the activation of cellular phospholipase A2. FEBS Lett. 1992;309(2):190–2.

92. Jaffer OA, Carter AB, Sanders PN, Dibbern ME, Winters CJ, Murthy S, et al. Mitochondrial-targeted antioxidant therapy decreases transforming growth factor-β-mediated collagen production in a murine asthma model. Am J Respir Cell Mol Biol. 2015;52(1):106–15.

93. Beghè B, Rabe KF, Fabbri LM. Phosphodiesterase-4 inhibitor therapy for lung diseases. Am J Respir Crit Care Med. 2013;188(3):271–8.

94. Diamant Z, Spina D. PDE4-inhibitors: a novel, targeted therapy for obstructive airways disease. Pulm Pharmacol Ther. 2011;24(4):353–60.

95. Michalski JM, Golden G, Ikari J, Rennard SI. PDE4: a novel target in the treatment of chronic obstructive pulmonary disease. Clin Pharmacol Ther. 2012;91(1):134–42.

96. Oba Y, Lone NA. Efficacy and safety of roflumilast in patients with chronic obstructive pulmonary disease: a systematic review and meta analysis. Ther Adv Respir Dis. 2013;7(1):13–24.

97. Gauvreau GM, Boulet LP, Schmid-Wirlitsch C, Côté J, Duong M, Killian KJ, et al. Roflumilast attenuates allergen-induced inflammation in mild asthmatic subjects. Respir Res. 2011;12:140.

98. Harbinson PL, MacLeod D, Hawksworth R, O'Toole S, Sullivan PJ, Heath P, et al. The effect of a novel orally active selective PDE4 isoenzyme inhibitor (CDP840) on allergen-induced responses in asthmatic subjects. Eur Respir J. 1997;10(5):1008–14.

99. van Schalkwyk E, Strydom K, Williams Z, Venter L, Leichtl S, Schmid-Wirlitsch C, et al. Roflumilast, an oral, once daily phosphodiesterase 4 inhibitor, attenuates allergen-induced asthmatic reactions. J Allergy Clin Immunol. 2005;116(2):292–8.

100. Louw C, Williams Z, Venter L, Leichtl S, Schmid-Wirlitsch C, Bredenbroker D, et al. Roflumilast, a phosphodiesterase 4 inhibitor, reduces airway hyperresponsiveness after allergen challenge. Respiration. 2007;74(4):411–7.

101. Gauvreau GM, Evans MY. Allergen inhalation challenge: a human model of asthma exacerbation. Contrib Microbiol. 2007;14:21–32.

102. Timmer W, Leclerc V, Birraux G, Neuhäuser M, Hatzelmann A, Bethke T, et al. The new phosphodiesterase 4 inhibitor roflumilast is efficacious in exercise-induced asthma and leads to suppression of LPS-stimulated TNF-alpha ex vivo. J Clin Pharmacol. 2002;42(3):297–303.

103. Bousquet J, Aubier M, Sastre J, Izquierdo JL, Adler LM, Hofbauer P, et al. Comparison of roflumilast, an oral anti-inflammatory, with beclomethasone dipropionate in the treatment of persistent asthma. Allergy. 2006;61(1):72–8.

104. Houslay MD, Schafer P, Zhang KY. Keynote review: phosphodiesterase-4 as a therapeutic target. Drug Discov Today. 2005;10(22):1503–19.

105. Banner KH, Press NJ. Dual PDE3/4 inhibitors as therapeutic agents for chronic obstructive pulmonary disease. Br J Pharmacol. 2009;157(6):892–906.

106. Ron D, Walter P. Signal integration in the endoplasmic reticulum unfolded protein response. Nat Rev Mol Cell Biol. 2007;8(7):519–29.

107. Kim I, Xu W, Reed JC. Cell death and endoplasmic reticulum stress: disease relevance and therapeutic opportunities. Nat Rev Drug Discov. 2008;7(12):1013–30.

108. Toth A, Nickson P, Mandl A, Bannister ML, Toth K, Erhardt P, et al. Endoplasmic reticulum stress as a novel therapeutic target in heart diseases. Cardiovasc Hematol Disord Drug Targets. 2007;7(3):205–18.

109. Kelsen SG, Duan X, Ji R, Perez O, Liu C, Merali S, et al. Cigarette smoke induces an unfolded protein response in the human lung: a proteomic approach. Am J Respir Cell Mol Biol. 2008;38(5):541–50.

110. Poppek D, Grune T. Proteasomal defense of oxidative protein modifications. Antioxid Redox Signal. 2006;8(1–2):173–84.

111. Osorio F, Lambrecht B, Janssens S. The UPR and lung disease. Semin Immunopathol. 2013;35(3):293–306.

112. Wei J, Rahman S, Ayaub EA, Dickhout JG, Ask K. Protein misfolding and endoplasmic reticulum stress in chronic lung disease. Chest. 2013;143(4):1098–105.

113. Ozcan U, Yilmaz E, Ozcan L, Furuhashi M, Vaillancourt E, Smith RO, et al. Chemical chaperones reduce ER stress and restore glucose homeostasis in a mouse model of type 2 diabetes. Science. 2006;313(5790):1137–40.

114. Kars M, Yang L, Gregor MF, Mohammed BS, Pietka TA, Finck BN, et al. Tauroursodeoxycholic acid may improve liver and muscle but not adipose tissue insulin sensitivity in obese men and women. Diabetes. 2010;59(8):1899–905.

115. Zode GS, Kuehn MH, Nishimura DY, Searby CC, Mohan K, Grozdanic SD, et al. Reduction of ER stress via a chemical chaperone prevents disease phenotypes in a mouse model of primary open angle glaucoma. J Clin Invest. 2011;121(9):3542–53.

116. Sorrentino SA, Besler C, Rohrer L, Meyer M, Heinrich K, Bahlmann FH, et al. Endothelial-vasoprotective effects of high-density lipoprotein are impaired in patients with type 2 diabetes mellitus but are improved after extended-release niacin therapy. Circulation. 2010;121(1):110–22.

117. Mily A, Rekha RS, Kamal SM, Akhtar E, Sarker P, Rahim Z, et al. Oral intake of phenylbutyrate with or without vitamin D3 upregulates the cathelicidin LL-37 in human macrophages: a dose finding study for treatment of tuberculosis. BMC Pulm Med. 2013;13:23.

118. Klein S. Washington University School of Medicine. Effect of endoplasmic reticulum stress on metabolic function (TUDCA/PBA). 1999. http://clinicaltrials.gov/show/NCT00004451. Updated 29 Nov 2005; Accessed 6 May 2017.

119. Rubenstein R. The Children's Hospital of Philadelphia. Phenylbutyrate/genistein duotherapy in delta F508-heterozygotes (for cystic fibrosis). 1999. http://clinicaltrials.gov/show/NCT000164744. Updated 23 Jun 2005; Accessed 6 May 2017.

120. Makhija L, Krishnan V, Rehman R, Chakraborty S, Maity S, Mabalirajan U, et al. Chemical chaperones mitigate experimental asthma by attenuating endoplasmic reticulum stress. Am J Respir Cell Mol Biol. 2014;50(5):923–31.

121. MacGlashan DW, Bochner BS, Adelman DC, Jardieu PM, Togias A, McKenzie-White J, et al. Down-regulation of FcεRI expression on human basophils during in vivo treatment of atopic patients with anti-IgE antibody. J Immunol. 1997;158(3):1438–45.

122. Holgate S, Casale T, Wenzel S, Bousquet J, Deniz Y, Reisner C, et al. The anti-inflammatory effects of omalizumab confirm the central role of IgE in allergic inflammation. J Allergy Clin Immunol. 2005;115(3):459–65.

123. Djukanovic R, Wilson SJ, Kraft M, Jarjour NN, Steel M, Chung KF, et al. Effects of treatment with anti-immunoglobulin E antibody omalizumab on airway inflammation in allergic asthma. Am J Respir Crit Care Med. 2004;170(6):583–93.

124. Chipps BE, Lanier B, Milgrom H, Deschildre A, Hedlin G, Szefler SJ, et al. Omalizumab in children with uncontrolled allergic asthma: review of clinical trial and real-world experience. J Allergy Clin Immunol. 2017;139(5):1431–44.

125. Chung KF, Wenzel SE, Brozek JL, Bush A, Castro M, Sterk PJ, et al. International ERS/ATS guidelines on definition, evaluation and treatment of severe asthma. Eur Respir J. 2014;43(2):343–73.

126. Agrawal DK, Shao Z. Pathogenesis of allergic airway inflammation. Curr Allergy Asthma Rep. 2010;10:39–48.

127. Humbert M, Busse W, Hanania NA, Lowe PJ, Canvin J, Erpenbeck VJ, et al. Omalizumab in asthma: an update on recent developments. J Allergy Clin Immunol Pract. 2014;2(5):525–36.e1.

128. Fahy JV, Fleming HE, Wong HH, Liu JT, Su JQ, Reimann J, et al. The effect of an anti-IgE monoclonal antibody on the early- and late-phase responses to allergen inhalation in asthmatic subjects. Am J Respir Crit Care Med. 1997;155(6):1828–34.

129. Samitas K, Delimpoura V, Zervas E, Gaga M. Anti-IgE treatment, airway inflammation and remodelling in severe allergic asthma: current knowledge and future perspectives. Eur Respir Rev. 2015;24(138):594–601.

130. Teach SJ, Gill MA, Togias A, Sorkness CA, Arbes SJ Jr, Calatroni A, et al. Preseasonal treatment with either omalizumab or an inhaled corticosteroid boost to prevent fall asthma exacerbations. J Allergy Clin Immunol. 2015;136(6):1476–85.

131. Moffatt MF, Gut IG, Demenais F, Strachan DP, Bouzigon E, Heath S, et al. A large-scale, consortium-based genome wide association study of asthma. N Engl J Med. 2010;363(13):1211–21.

132. Busse WW, Morgan WJ, Gergen PJ, Mitchell HE, Gern JE, Liu AH, et al. Randomized trial of omalizumab (anti-IgE) for asthma in inner-city children. N Engl J Med. 2011;364(11):1005–15.

133. Hanania NA, Alpan O, Hamilos DL, Condemi JJ, Reyes-Rivera I, Zhu J, et al. Omalizumab in severe allergic asthma inadequately controlled with standard therapy: a randomized trial. Ann Intern Med. 2011;154(9):573–82.

134. Rodrigo GJ, Neffen H, Castro-Rodriguez JA. Efficacy and safety of subcutaneous omalizumab vs placcbo as add on therapy to corticosteroids for children and adults with asthma: a systematic review. Chest. 2011;139(1):28–35.

135. US Food and Drug Administration (FDA). Xolair (omalizumab) US prescribing information. 2014. www.accessdata.fda.gov/drugsatfda_docs/label/2014/103976s5161lbl.pdf. Accessed 23 Nov 2016.

136. European Medicines Agency (EMA). Xolair (omalizumab) summary of product characteristics. 2016. http://www.ema.europa.eu/docs/en_GB/document_library/EPAR_-_Product_Information/human/000606/WC500057298.pdf. Accessed 23 Nov 2016.

137. National Institute for Health and Care Excellence (NICE). Omalizumab for the treatment of severe persistent allergic asthma in children aged 6–11. 2010. https://www.nice.org.uk/guidance/ta201. Accessed 23 Nov 2016.

138. National Institute for Health and Care Excellence (NICE). Omalizumab for treating severe persistent allergic asthma (technology appraisal guidance). 2013. www.nice.org.uk/guidance/ta278. Accessed 31 May 2016.

139. Papadopoulos NG, Arakawa H, Carlsen KH, Custovic A, Gern J, Lemanske R, et al. International consensus on (ICON) pediatric asthma. Allergy. 2012;67(8):976–97.

140. National Asthma Education and Prevention Program. Third Expert Panel on the Diagnosis and Management of Asthma. Expert panel report 3: guidelines for the diagnosis and management of asthma. Bethesda, MD: National Heart, Lung, and Blood Institute; 2007.

141. Arm JP, Bottoli I, Skerjanec A, Floch D, Groenewegen A, Maahs S, et al. Pharmacokinetics, pharmacodynamics and safety of QGE031 (ligelizumab), a novel high-affinity anti-IgE antibody, in atopic subjects. Clin Exp Allergy. 2014;44(11):1371–85.

142. Maes T, Joos GF, Brusselle GG. Targeting interleukin-4 in asthma: lost in translation? Am J Respir Cell Mol Biol. 2012;47(3):261–70.

143. Grunig G, Warnock M, Wakil AE, Venkayya R, Brombacher F, Rennick DM, et al. Requirement for IL-13 independently of IL-4 in experimental asthma. Science. 1998;282(5397):2261–3.

144. Wills-Karp M, Luyimbazi J, Xu X, Schofield B, Neben TY, Karp CL, et al. Interleukin-13: central mediator of allergic asthma. Science. 1998;282(5397):2258–61.

145. Chatila TA. Interleukin-4 receptor signaling pathways in asthma pathogenesis. Trends Mol Med. 2004;10(10):493–9.

146. Wenzel S, Wilbraham D, Fuller R, Getz EB, Longphre M. Effect of an nterleukin-4 variant on late phase asthmatic response to allergen challenge in asthmatic patients: results of two phase 2a studies. Lancet. 2007;370(9596):1422–31.

147. Slager RE, Otulana BA, Hawkins GA, Yen YP, Peters SP, Wenzel SE, et al. IL-4 receptor polymorphisms predict reduction in asthma exacerbations during response to an anti-IL-4 receptor a antagonist. J Allergy Clin Immunol. 2012;130(2):516–22. e4.

148. Corren J, Busse W, Meltzer EO, Mansfield L, Bensch G, Fahrenholz J, et al. A randomized, controlled, phase 2 study of AMG 317, an IL- 4Ralpha antagonist, in patients with asthma. Am J Respir Crit Care Med. 2010;181(8):788–96.

149. Wenzel S, Ford L, Pearlman D, Spector S, Sher L, Skobieranda F, et al. Dupilumab in persistent asthma with elevated eosinophil levels. N Engl J Med. 2013;368(26):2455–66.

150. Wenzel S, Castro M, Corren J, Maspero J, Wang L, Zhang B, et al. Dupilumab efficacy and safety in adults with uncontrolled persistent asthma despite use of medium-to-high-dose inhaled corticosteroids plus a long-acting β2 agonist: a randomized double-blind placebo-controlled pivotal phase 2b dose-ranging trial. Lancet. 2016;388(10039):31–44.

151. Corren J, Lemanske RF, Hanania NA, Korenblat PE, Parsey MV, Arron JR, et al. Lebrikizumab treatment in adults with asthma. N Engl J Med. 2011;365(12):1088–98.

152. Piper E, Brightling C, Niven R, Oh C, Faggioni R, Poon K, et al. A phase II placebo-controlled study of tralokinumab in moderate-to-severe asthma. Eur Respir J. 2013;41(2):330–8.

153. DeBoever EH, Ashman C, Cahn AP, Locantore NW, Overend P, Pouliquen IJ, et al. Efficacy and safety of an anti-IL-13 mAb in patients with severe asthma: a randomized trial. J Allergy Clin Immunol. 2014;133(4):989–96.

154. Hanania NA, Korenblat P, Chapman KR, Bateman ED, Kopecky P, Paggiaro P, et al. Efficacy and safety of lebrikizumab in patients with uncontrolled asthma (LAVOLTA I and LAVOLTA II): replicate, phase 3, randomised, double-blind, placebo-controlled trials. Lancet Respir Med. 2016;4(10):781–96.

155. Brightling CE, Chanez P, Leigh R, O'Byrne PM, Korn S, She D, et al. Efficacy and safety of tralokinumab in patients with severe uncontrolled asthma: a randomised, double-blind, placebo-controlled, phase 2b trial. Lancet Respir Med. 2015;3(9):692–701.

156. Clutterbuck EJ, Hirst EM, Sanderson CJ. Human interleukin-5 (IL-5) regulates the production of eosinophils in human bone marrow cultures: comparison and interaction with IL-1, IL-3, IL-6, and GMCSF. Blood. 1989;73(6):1504–12.

157. Licona-Limon P, Kim LK, Palm NW, Flavell RA. TH2, allergy and group 2 innate lymphoid cells. Nat Immunol. 2013;14(6):536–42.

158. Holtzman MJ, Byers DE, Alexander-Brett J, Wang X. The role of airway epithelial cells and innate immune cells in chronic respiratory disease. Nat Rev Immunol. 2014;14(10):686–98.

159. Bernink JH, Germar K, Spits H. The role of ILC2 in pathology of type 2 inflammatory diseases. Curr Opin Immunol. 2014;31:115–20.

160. Russell R, Brightling CE. Anti-IL-5 for severe asthma: aiming high to achieve success. Chest. 2016;150(4):766–8.

161. Flood-Page P, Swenson C, Faiferman I, Matthews J, Williams M, Brannick L, et al. A study to evaluate safety and efficacy of mepolizumab in patients with moderate persistent asthma. Am J Respir Crit Care Med. 2007;176(11):1062–71.

162. Leckie MJ, ten Brinke A, Khan J, Diamant Z, O'Connor BJ, Walls CM, et al. Effects of an interleukin-5 blocking monoclonal antibody on eosinophils, airway hyper-responsiveness, and the late asthmatic response. Lancet. 2000;356(9248):2144–8.

163. Pavord ID, Korn S, Howarth P, Bleecker ER, Buhl R, Keene ON, et al. Mepolizumab for severe eosinophilic asthma (DREAM): a multicentre, double-blind, placebo-controlled trial. Lancet. 2012;380(9842):651–9.

164. Haldar P, Brightling CE, Hargadon B, Gupta S, Monteiro W, Sousa A, et al. Mepolizumab and exacerbations of refractory eosinophilic asthma. N Engl J Med. 2009;360(10):973–84.

165. Nair P, Pizzichini MM, Kjarsgaard M, Kjarsgaard M, Inman MD, Efthimiadis A, et al. Mepolizumab for prednisone-dependent asthma with sputum eosinophilia. N Engl J Med. 2009;360(10):985–93.

166. Ortega HG, Liu MC, Pavord ID, Brusselle GG, FitzGerald JM, Chetta A, et al. Mepolizumab treatment in patients with severe eosinophilic asthma. N Engl J Med. 2014;371(13):1198–207.

167. Bel EH, Wenzel SE, Thompson PJ, Prazma CM, Keene ON, Yancey SW, et al. Oral glucocorticoid-sparing effect of mepolizumab in eosinophilic asthma. N Engl J Med. 2014;371(13):1189–97.

168. Castro M, Mathur S, Hargreave F, Boulet LP, Xie F, Young J, et al. Reslizumab for poorly controlled, eosinophilic asthma: a randomized, placebo-controlled study. Am J Respir Crit Care Med. 2011;184(10):1125–32.

169. Castro M, Zangrilli J, Wechsler ME, Bateman ED, Brusselle GG, Bardin P, et al. Reslizumab for inadequately controlled asthma with elevated blood eosinophil counts: results from two multicentre, parallel,

double-blind, randomised, placebo-controlled, phase 3 trials. Lancet Respir Med. 2015;3(5):355–66.

170. Kolbeck R, Kozhich A, Koike M, Peng L, Andersson CK, Damschroder MM, et al. MEDI-563, a humanized anti-IL-5 receptor alpha mAb with enhanced antibody-dependent cell-mediated cytotoxicity function. J Allergy Clin Immunol. 2010;125(6):1344–53.e2.

171. FitzGerald JM, Bleecker ER, Nair P, Korn S, Ohta K, Lommatzsch M, et al. Benralizumab, an anti-interleukin-5 receptor α monoclonal antibody, as add-on treatment for patients with severe, uncontrolled, eosinophilic asthma (CALIMA): a randomised, double-blind, placebo-controlled phase 3 trial. Lancet. 2016;388(10056):2128–41.

172. Bleecker ER, FitzGerald JM, Chanez P, Papi A, Weinstein SF, Barker P, et al. Efficacy and safety of benralizumab for patients with severe asthma uncontrolled with high-dosage inhaled corticosteroids and long-acting β2-agonists (SIROCCO): a randomised, multicentre, placebo-controlled phase 3 trial. Lancet. 2016;388(10056):2115–27.

173. Castro M, Wenzel SE, Bleecker ER, Pizzichini E, Kuna P, Busse WW, et al. Benralizumab, an anti-interleukin 5 receptor α monoclonal antibody, versus placebo for uncontrolled eosinophilic asthma: a phase 2b randomized dose-ranging study. Lancet Respir Med. 2014;2(11):879–90.

174. Toba K, Koike T, Shibata A, Hashimoto S, Takahashi M, Masuko M, et al. Novel technique for the direct flow cytofluorometric analysis of human basophils in unseparated blood and bone marrow, and the characterization of phenotype and peroxidase of human basophils. Cytometry. 1999;35(3):249–59.

175. Laviolette M, Gossage DL, Gauvreau G, Leigh R, Olivenstein R, Katial R, et al. Effects of benralizumab on airway eosinophils in asthmatic patients with sputum eosinophilia. J Allergy Clin Immunol. 2013;132(5):1086–96.e5.

176. Liu YJ, Soumelis V, Watanabe N, Ito T, Wang YH, Malefyt Rde W, et al. TSLP: an epithelial cell cytokine that regulates T cell diff erentiation by conditioning dendritic cell maturation. Annu Rev Immunol. 2007;25:193–219.

177. Ying S, O'Connor B, Ratoff J, Meng Q, Fang C, Cousins D, et al. Expression and cellular provenance of thymic stromal lymphopoietin and chemokines in patients with severe asthma and chronic obstructive pulmonary disease. J Immunol. 2008;181(4):2790–8.

178. Gauvreau GM, O'Byrne PM, Boulet LP, Wang Y, Cockcroft D, Bigler J, et al. Effects of an anti-TSLP antibody on allergen-induced asthmatic responses. N Engl J Med. 2014;370(22):2102–10.

179. MedImmune LLC. A phase 2 randomized, double-blind, placebo-controlled study to evaluate the efficacy and safety of MEDI9929 in adult subjects with inadequately controlled, severe asthma. 2013. http://clinicaltrials.gov/show/NCT02054130. Updated 13 Apr 2017; Accessed 6 May 2017.

180. Porsbjerg C. Effects of anti-TSLP on airway hyper-responsiveness and mast cell phenotype in asthma—a randomized double-blind, placebo-controlled trial of MEDI9929. 2016. http://clinicaltrials.gov/show/NCT02698501. Updated 3 Jan 2017; Accessed 6 May 2017.

181. Robinson DS, Campbell DA, Barnes PJ. Addition of an anti-leukotriene to therapy in chronic severe asthma in a clinic setting: a double-blind, randomised, placebo-controlled study. Lancet. 2001;357(9273):2007–11.

182. Leff JA, Busse WW, Pearlman D, Bronsky EA, Kemp J, Hendeles L, et al. Montelukast, a leukotriene-receptor antagonist, for the treatment of mild asthma and exercise-induced bronchoconstriction. N Engl J Med. 1998;339(3):147–52.

183. Ohnishi H, Miyahara N, Gelfand EW. The role of leukotriene B(4) in allergic diseases. Allergol Int 2008;57(4):291–8.

184. Tager AM, Luster AD. BLT1 and BLT2: the leukotriene B(4) receptors. Prostaglandins Leukot Essent Fatty Acids. 2003;69(2–3):123–34.

185. Rao NL, Riley JP, Banie H, Xue X, Sun B, Crawford S, et al. Leukotriene A(4) hydrolase inhibition attenuates allergic airway inflammation and hyper-responsiveness. Am J Respir Crit Care Med. 2010;181(9):899–907.

186. Cho KJ, Seo JM, Shin Y, Yoo MH, Park CS, Lee SH, et al. Blockade of airway inflammation and hyper-responsiveness by inhibition of BLT2, a low-affinity leukotriene B4 receptor. Am J Respir Cell Mol Biol. 2010;42(3):294–303.

187. Aronson JK. Side effects of drugs annual: a worldwide yearly survey of new data and trends in adverse drug reactions and interactions. Side Effects Drugs Annu. 2010;32:1–1004.

188. Grant GE, Rokach J, Powell WS. 5-Oxo-ETE and the OXE receptor. Prostaglandins Other Lipid Mediat. 2009;89(3–4):98–104.

189. Kent SE, Boyce M, Diamant Z, Singh D, O'Connor BJ, Saggu PS, et al. The 5-lipoxygenase-activating protein inhibitor, GSK2190915, attenuates the early and late responses to inhaled allergen in mild asthma. Clin Exp Allergy. 2013;43(2):177–86.

190. Pettipher R, Hansel TT, Armer R. Antagonism of the prostaglandin D2 receptors DP1 and CRTH2 as an approach to treat allergic diseases. Nat Rev Drug Discov. 2007;6(4):313–25.

191. Peters MC, Mekonnen ZK, Yuan S, Bhakta NR, Woodruff PG, Fahy JV, et al. Measures of gene expression in sputum cells can identify TH2-high and TH2-low subtypes of asthma. J Allergy Clin Immunol. 2014;133(2):388–94.

192. Balzar S, Fajt ML, Comhair SA, Erzurum SC, Bleecker E, Busse WW, et al. Mast cell phenotype, location, and activation in severe asthma: data from the severe asthma research program. Am J Respir Crit Care Med. 2011;183(3):299–309.

193. Chung KF. Targeting the interleukin pathway in the treatment of asthma. Lancet. 2015;386(9998):1086–96.

194. Barnes N, Pavord I, Chuchalin A, Bell J, Hunter M, Lewis T, et al. A randomized, double-blind, placebo-controlled study of the CRTH2 antagonist OC000459 in moderate persistent asthma. Clin Exp Allergy. 2012;42(1):38–48.

195. Busse WW, Wenzel SE, Meltzer EO, Kerwin EM, Liu MC, Zhang N, et al. Safety and efficacy of the prostaglandin D2 receptor antagonist AMG 853 in asthmatic patients. Allergy Clin Immunol. 2013;131(2):339–45.

196. Hall IP, Fowler AV, Gupta A, Tetzlaff K, Nivens MC, Sarno M, et al. Efficacy of BI 671800, an oral CRTH2 antagonist, in poorly controlled asthma as sole controller and in the presence of inhaled corticosteroid treatment. Pulm Pharmacol Ther. 2015;32:37–44.

197. Berair R, Gonem S, Singapuri A, Hartley R, Laurencin M, Bacher G, et al. Effect of QAW039, an oral prostaglandin D2 receptor (DP2/CrTh2) antagonist upon sputum and bronchial eosinophilic inflammation and clinical outcomes in treatment-resistant asthma: a phase 2a randomised placebo-controlled trial. Am J Respir Crit Care Med. 2015;191:A6361.

198. Lodowski DT, Palczewski K. Chemokine receptors and other G protein coupled receptors. Curr Opin HIV AIDS. 2009;4(2):88–95.

199. Gauvreau GM, Boulet LP, Cockcroft DW, Baatjes A, Cote J, Deschesnes F, et al. Antisense therapy against CCR3 and the common beta chain attenuates allergen induced eosinophilic responses. Am J Respir Crit Care Med. 2008;177(9):952–8.

200. Tomankova T, Kriegova E, Liu M. Chemokine receptors and their therapeutic opportunities in diseased lung: far beyond leukocyte trafficking. Am J Physiol Lung Cell Mol Physiol. 2015;308(7):L603–18.

201. Antoniu SA. Mogamulizumab, a humanized mAb against C-C chemokine receptor 4 for the potential treatment of T-cell lymphomas and asthma. Curr Opin Mol Ther. 2010;12(6):770–9.

202. Solari R, Pease JE. Targeting chemokine receptors in disease—a case study of CCR4. Eur J Pharmacol. 2015;763(Pt B):169–77.

203. Cahn A, Hodgson S, Wilson R, Robertson J, Watson J, Beerahee M, et al. Safety, tolerability, pharmacokinetics and pharmacodynamics of GSK2239633, a CC-chemokine receptor 4 antagonist, in healthy male subjects: results from an open-label and from a randomised study. BMC Pharmacol Toxicol. 2013;14:14.

204. Kips JC, Tavernier J, Pauwels RA. Tumor necrosis factor causes bronchial hyperresponsiveness in rats. Am Rev Respir Dis. 1992;145(2 Pt 1):332–6.

205. Holgate ST, Noonan M, Chanez P, Busse W, Dupont L, Pavord I, et al. Efficacy and safety of etanercept in moderate-to-severe asthma: a randomised, controlled trial. Eur Respir J. 2011;37(6):1352–9.

206. Proudfoot AE, Power CA, Schwarz MK. Anti-chemokine small molecule drugs: a promising future? Expert Opin Investig Drugs. 2010;19(3):345–55.

207. Erin EM, Leaker BR, Nicholson GC, Tan AJ, Green LM, Neighbour H, et al. The effects of a monoclonal antibody directed against tumor necrosis factor-alpha in asthma. Am J Respir Crit Care Med. 2006;174(7):753–62.

208. Wenzel SE, Barnes PJ, Bleecker ER, Bousquet J, Busse W, Dahlén SE, et al. A randomized, double-blind, placebo-controlled study of tumor necrosis factor-alpha blockade in severe persistent asthma. Am J Respir Crit Care Med. 2009;179(7):549–58.

209. Park SJ, Lee KS, Kim SR, Min KH, Choe YH, Moon H, et al. Peroxisome proliferator-activated receptor gamma agonist down-regulates IL-17 expression in a murine model of allergic airway inflammation. J Immunol. 2009;183(5):3259–67.

210. Molet S, Hamid Q, Davoine F, Nutku E, Taha R, Pagé N, et al. IL-17 is increased in asthmatic airways and induces human bronchial fibroblasts to produce cytokines. J Allergy Clin Immunol. 2001;108(3):430–8.

211. Barczyk A, Pierzchala W, Sozañska E. Interleukin-17 in sputum correlates with airway hyperresponsiveness to methacholine. Respir Med. 2003;97(6):726–33.

212. Sun Y-C, Zhou Q-T, Yao W-Z. Sputum interleukin-17 is increased and associated with airway neutrophilia in patients with severe asthma. Chin Med J. 2005;118(11):953–6.

213. Bullens DM, Truyen E, Coteur L, Dilissen E, Hellings PW, Dupont LJ, et al. IL-17 mRNA in sputum of asthmatic patients: linking T cell driven inflammation and granulocytic influx? Respir Res. 2006;7:135.

214. Rickel EA, Siegel LA, Yoon BR, Rottman JB, Kugler DG, Swart DA, et al. Identification of functional roles for both IL-17RB and IL-17RA in mediating IL-25-induced activities. J Immunol. 2008;181(6):4299–310.

215. Busse WW, Holgate S, Kerwin E, Chon Y, Feng J, Lin J, et al. Randomized, double-blind, placebo-controlled study of brodalumab, a human anti-IL-17 receptor monoclonal antibody, in moderate to severe asthma. Am J Respir Crit Care Med. 2013;188(11):1294–302.

216. Besnard AG, Guillou N, Tschopp J, Erard F, Couillin I, Iwakura Y, et al. NLRP3 inflammasome is required in murine asthma in the absence of aluminum adjuvant. Allergy. 2011;66(8):1047–57.

217. Kool M, Pétrilli V, De Smedt T, Rolaz A, Hammad H, van Nimwegen M, et al. Cutting edge: alum adjuvant stimulates inflammatory dendritic cells through activation of the NALP3 inflammasome. J Immunol. 2008;181(6):3755–9.

218. Gregory LG, Lloyd CM. Orchestrating house dust mite-associated allergy in the lung. Trends Immunol. 2011;32(9):402–11.

219. Kim RY, Pinkerton JW, Essilfie AT, Robertson AA, Baines KJ, Brown AC, et al. Role for NLRP3 inflammasome-mediated, IL-1β-dependent responses

in severe, steroid-resistant asthma. Am J Respir Crit Care Med 2017. doi:10.1164/rccm.201609-1830OC.

220. Kuo CS, Pavlidis S, Loza M, Baribaud F, Rowe A, Pandis I, et al. T-helper cell type 2 (Th2) and non-Th2 molecular phenotypes of asthma using sputum transcriptomics in U-BIOPRED. Eur Respir J. 2017;49(2):pii: 1602135.

221. Holz O, Khalilieh S, Ludwig-Sengpiel A, Watz H, Stryszak P, Soni P, et al. SCH527123, a novel CXCR2 antagonist, inhibits ozone-induced neutrophilia in healthy subjects. Eur Respir J. 2010;35(3):564–70.

222. Nair P, Gaga M, Zervas E, Alagha K, Hargreave FE, O'Byrne PM, et al. Safety and efficacy of a CXCR2 antagonist in patients with severe asthma and sputum neutrophils: a randomized, placebo-controlled clinical trial. Clin Exp Allergy. 2012;42(7):097–1103.

223. de Oliveira S, Rosowski EE, Huttenlocher A. Neutrophil migration in infection and wound repair: going forward in reverse. Nat Rev Immunol. 2016;16(6):378–91.

224. Moss RB. Treatment options in severe fungal asthma and allergic bronchopulmonary aspergillosis. Eur Respir J. 2014;43(5):1487–500.

225. Denning DW, Van Wye JE, Lewiston NJ, Stevens DA. Adjunctive therapy of allergic bronchopulmonary aspergillosis with itraconazole. Chest. 1991;100(3):813–9.

226. Pacheco A, Martin JA, Cuevas M. Serologic response to itraconazole in allergic bronchopulmonary aspergillosis. Chest. 1993;103(3):980–1.

227. Germaud P, Tuchais E. Allergic bronchopulmonary aspergillosis treated with itraconazole. Chest. 1995;107(3):883.

228. Salez F, Brichet A, Desurmont S, Grosbois JM, Wallaert B, Tonnel AB, et al. Effects of itraconazole therapy in allergic bronchopulmonary aspergillosis. Chest. 1999;116(6):1658–65.

229. Stevens DA, Schwartz HJ, Lee JY, Moskovitz BL, Jerome DC, Catanzaro A, et al. A randomized trial of itraconazole in allergic bronchopulmonary aspergillosis. N Engl J Med. 2000;342(11):756–62.

230. Wark PA, Hensley MJ, Saltos N, Boyle MJ, Toneguzzi RC, Epid GD, et al. Anti inflammatory effect of itraconazole in stable allergic bronchopulmonary aspergillosis: a randomized controlled trial. J Allergy Clin Immunol. 2003;111(5):952–7.

231. Wark P. Pathogenesis of allergic bronchopulmonary aspergillosis and an evidence-based review of azoles in treatment. Respir Med. 2004;98(10):915–23.

232. Wark PA, Gibson PG, Wilson AJ. Azoles for allergic bronchopulmonary aspergillosis associated with asthma. Cochrane Database Syst Rev. 2004;3:CD001108.

233. Denning DW, O'Driscoll BR, Powell G, Chew F, Atherton GT, Vyas A, et al. Randomized controlled trial of oral antifungal treatment for severe asthma with fungal sensitization: the Fungal Asthma Sensitization Trial (FAST) study. Am J Respir Crit Care Med. 2009;179(1):11–8.

234. Vicencio AG, Chupp GL, Tsirilakis K, He X, Kessel A, Nandalike K, et al. CHIT1 mutations: genetic risk factor for severe asthma with fungal sensitization? Pediatrics. 2010;126(4):e982–5.

235. Vicencio AG, Muzumdar H, Tsirilakis K, Kessel A, Nandalike K, Goldman DL, et al. Severe asthma with fungal sensitization in a child: response to itraconazole therapy. Pediatrics. 2010;125(5):e1255–8.

236. Proesmans M, Vermeulen F, Vreys M, De Boeck K. Use of nebulized amphotericin B in the treatment of allergic bronchopulmonary aspergillosis in cystic fibrosis. Int J Pediatr. 2010;2010:376287.

237. Hayes D Jr, Murphy BS, Lynch JE, Feola DJ. Aerosolized amphotericin for the treatment of allergic bronchopulmonary aspergillosis. Pediatr Pulmonol. 2010;45(11):1145–8.

238. Metz G, Kraft M. Effects of atypical infections with mycoplasma and chlamydia on asthma. Immunol Allergy Clin N Am. 2010;30(4):575–85.

239. Kraft M, Torvik JA, Trudeau JB, Wenzel SE, Martin RJ. Theophylline: potential antiinflammatory effects in nocturnal asthma. J Allergy Clin Immunol. 1996 Jun;97(6):1242–6.

240. Sutherland ER, King TS, Icitovic N, Ameredes BT, Bleecker E, Boushey HA, et al. A trial of clarithromycin for the treatment of suboptimally controlled asthma. J Allergy Clin Immunol. 2010;126(4):747–53.

241. Altenburg J, de Graaff CS, Stienstra Y, Sloos JH, van Haren EH, Koppers RJ, et al. Effect of azithromycin maintenance treatment on infectious exacerbations among patients with non-cystic fibrosis bronchiectasis: the BAT randomized controlled trial. JAMA. 2013;309(12):1251–9.

242. Brusselle GG, Vanderstichele C, Jordens P, Deman R, Slabbynck H, Ringoet V, et al. Azithromycin for prevention of exacerbations in severe asthma (AZISAST): a multicentre randomised double-blind placebo-controlled trial. Thorax. 2013;68(4):322–9.

243. Lohia S, Schlosser RJ, Soler ZM. Impact of intranasal corticosteroids on asthma outcomes in allergic rhinitis: a meta-analysis. Allergy. 2013;68(5):569–79.

244. Johnston SL, Pattemore PK, Sanderson G, Smith S, Campbell MJ, Josephs LK, et al. The relationship between upper respiratory infections and hospital admissions for asthma: a time-trend analysis. Am J Respir Crit Care Med. 1996;154(3 Pt 1):654–60.

245. Corne JM, Marshall C, Smith S, Schreiber J, Sanderson G, Holgate ST, et al. Frequency, severity, and duration of rhinovirus infections in asthmatic and non-asthmatic individuals: a longitudinal cohort study. Lancet. 2002;359(9309):831–4.

246. Papadopoulos NG, Christodoulou I, Rohde G, Agache I, Almqvist C, Bruno A, et al. Viruses and bacteria in acute asthma exacerbations— a GA² LEN-DARE systematic review. Allergy. 2011;66(4):458–68.

247. Jackson DJ, Johnston SL. The role of viruses in acute exacerbations of asthma. J Allergy Clin Immunol. 2010;125(6):1178–87.

248. Bateman ED, Hurd SS, Barnes PJ, Bousquet J, Drazen JM, FitzGerald M, et al. Global strategy for asthma management and prevention: GINA executive summary. Eur Respir J. 2008;31(1):143–78.

249. Calışkan M, Bochkov YA, Kreiner-Møller E, Bønnelykke K, Stein MM, Du G, Bisgaard H, et al. Rhinovirus wheezing illness and genetic risk of childhood-onset asthma. N Engl J Med. 2013;368(15):1398–407.

250. Wark PA, Johnston SL, Bucchieri F, Powell R, Puddicombe S, Laza-Stanca V, et al. Asthmatic bronchial epithelial cells have a deficient innate immune response to infection with rhinovirus. J Exp Med. 2005;201(6):937–47.

251. Djukanović R, Harrison T, Johnston SL, Gabbay F, Wark P, Thomson NC, et al. The effect of inhaled IFN-β on worsening of asthma symptoms caused by viral infections. A randomized trial. Am J Respir Crit Care Med. 2014;190(2):145–54.

252. Holgate ST. Pathophysiology of asthma: what has our current understanding taught us about new therapeutic approaches? J Allergy Clin Immunol. 2011;128(3):495–505.

Non-pharmacologic Therapies for Severe Asthma

7

Yoon-Seok Chang

7.1 Education, Partnership, and Action Plan

It is always important to provide a proper education and to build a partnership in the management of severe asthma. Clinical outcome could be very dependent on the education and the partnership in severe asthma.

Inhalers such as inhaled corticosteroids, long-acting beta2 agonists, long-acting muscarinic receptor antagonists, and short-acting beta2 agonists are main treatment modalities of severe asthma. Inhalers are not like pills that patients simply swallow with water: they have to learn how to use inhalers properly. I had a patient who visited my clinic due to frequent admissions by exacerbated asthma. He had to visit the emergency room because of asthma exacerbation at least once a month for 4 months, which led to subsequent admissions for several days each time. After listening to his story, I investigated all the medications that he was taking at his first visit. Interestingly, he was taking a perfect list of medications for severe asthma: high-dose inhaled corti-

costeroid with a long-acting beta2 agonist, a long-acting muscarinic receptor antagonist, theophylline, and a leukotriene receptor antagonist. I simply checked his inhaler technique, which revealed the secret of the frequent exacerbations. He totally did not know how to use the inhalers. After learning how to use inhalers properly, his life changed dramatically. He could avoid further emergency visits or admissions! There are many examples like this including cases in athletes who had to give up their career because of severe asthma despite of medications, which turned out that it was because of their poor inhaler technique or poor adhesion. Of course, after a proper education and partnership, they could continue their loving sports with controlled asthma. It has been reported that many of asthma patients do not know how to use inhalers properly [1]. However, it is not just patients but also physicians. It has been reported that many general physicians do not know how to use inhalers properly, which addresses the importance of education on inhaler technique during the medical trainee courses [2, 3].

It is also important for patients to get the idea that asthma is a chronic inflammatory disease of the airway. Patients easily understand the meaning of "chronic disease" if you show the examples of chronic diseases such as diabetes mellitus or hypertension which need continued pharmacologic and non-pharmacologic treatment for the management. Showing the figures or video clips of underlying inflammation in severe asthma may impress patients: patients would understand that

Y.-S. Chang
Division of Allergy and Clinical Immunology, Department of Internal Medicine, Seoul National University Bundang Hospital, Seoul National University College of Medicine, Seongnam 13620, South Korea
e-mail: addchang@snu.ac.kr

their symptoms of dyspnea and wheezing are not just caused by bronchospasm but also by chronic airway inflammation which is the target of inhaled corticosteroid. The patients should be aware that they must keep regular medications including inhaled corticosteroid even after their symptoms disappear. They must understand the concept of management steps in asthma [4–6]. Especially for severe asthma, adherence is very important in the management. Poor adherence or stopping medications is one of the leading causes of visiting the emergency room due to acute asthma exacerbation [7]. Physicians should be aware that the patients does not normally wish to take regular medications for long term. This is true even for some patients with definite symptoms. Environmental factors such as inhalant allergens, smoking, indoor and outdoor air pollutions, and infections should also be considered in severe asthma patients (see next session). One of the key factors for successful education and partnership is education in self-management.

A written action plan is a very important strategy in self-management and should be provided to patients with severe asthma. It includes the daily action plan and the action plan for acute exacerbation of asthma [4–6]. Action plan shows how to recognize the loss of control and the severity of asthma: most of action plans show green (good), yellow (mild to moderate), and red (severe) zone according to the symptoms and peak flow meter. For example, in green zone, action plans show that the patient should take long-term control medications every day and show instructions such as how to prepare exercise or things to avoid. If the patient has one or more of the symptoms such as wheezing, chest tightness, cough, shortness of breath, waking up at night due to asthma symptoms, and the limitation of activities due to asthma symptoms or some decrease in peak flow, the action plans show that the patient is in yellow zone and show the instructions that the patient should take long-term control medicines and that the patient should increase or add some medicine within 1 h if the patient still has the symptoms or decreased peak flow. If the patient has urgent signs of severe asthma

Table 7.1 Suggested educational contents in severe asthma

Symptoms and signs of severe asthma
Prevalence of asthma and severe asthma
Socioeconomic burden of severe asthma
Cause and trigger factors
Mechanism and partnership: asthma is a chronic inflammatory airway disease
Avoidance: environmental control
Understanding the medications
How to use inhalers
How to exercise
Action plan according to symptoms and signs
Possible side effects
Comorbid conditions

exacerbation (severe dyspnea, difficulty in walking or talking due to dyspnea, cyanosis, severely decreased peak flow (e.g. less than 50% of personal best), the action plans will present the warning signs and advise to take prescribed rescue medicines, to ask for immediate help, or to call 911.

Asthma is a common allergic disease with high socioeconomic burden: although the proportion is small, severe asthma spends much more healthcare costs than mild to moderate asthma [8–10]. Education, partnership, and action plan are the key components of non-pharmacologic management in severe asthma. Suggested educational contents for severe asthma patients are summarized (Table 7.1).

7.2   Environmental Control

If asthma control is not achieved, it is always important to check the inhaler technique and adherence but also the environmental factors.

Inhalant allergens such as house dust mites, cat, dog, cockroach, fungi, and pollens can provoke acute exacerbations of asthma and contribute to the severity of asthma depending on the causative allergens of each patient. It is helpful to identify the causative allergens by skin prick test or the measurement of serum allergen-specific IgE, which should be interpreted with clinical correlation. In suspected cases, appropriate measures could be considered to eliminate or reduce the exposure to the causative allergens. As studies of individual aeroallergen avoidance strategies show that single interventions have limited or no benefit, a multifaceted approach is more likely to be effective if it addresses all the indoor asthma triggers. For house dust mite, a Cochrane review showed that chemical and physical methods of reducing exposure to house dust mite allergens at home (including acaricides, mattress covers, vacuum cleaning, heating, ventilation, freezing, washing, air filtration, and ionizers) were ineffective [5, 11].

Occupational allergens such as isocyanate and reactive dyes can also contribute to the development of severe asthma and should be evaluated in suspected cases [12–14]. Identification of the occupational asthma and the causative allergen is very important because early avoidance is strongly recommended.

Smoking can provoke acute asthma exacerbation but also severe asthma. It has been reported that smoking can reduce the lung function early in asthma and the response to medications, particularly inhaled corticosteroid [15]. Stop smoking and avoiding the exposure to smoking (passive smoking) are very important in the management of severe asthma.

Air pollution can provoke the aggravation of asthma. It has been reported that asthma-related morbidity and mortality could be increased due to air pollution [16, 17]. Particulate matter (PM), ozone (O_3), nitrogen oxides (NO_x), and SO2 are major outdoor air pollutants that contribute to increased susceptibility to respiratory infection [18, 19]. PM is a complex mixture of liquid droplets and extremely small particles, composed of organic and inorganic compounds [20]. PM_{10} is a PM less than 10 μm in aerodynamic diameter, which can penetrate conducting airways $PM_{2.5}$ is a PM less than 2.5 μm in aerodynamic diameter, which can penetrate into the gas-exchanging regions of the lung [20]. Sources of ambient PM include construction sites, smokestacks, fires, power plants, and automobiles; the main sources of indoor PM include ambient PM, tobacco smoke, cooking, and heating appliances. PM

causes lung inflammation and mucous secretion by acting on airway epithelial cells and alveolar macrophages and may lead to airway remodeling [20]. Some Asian countries such as China, Korea, and Japan suffer from Asian sand dust which originates from desert area of Mongolia and North China and which induces acute exacerbation of asthma [21]. Smoking, combustion pollutants, and volatile organic compounds such as formaldehyde and phthalate are examples of important indoor air pollution [16, 17]. For the quality of indoor air, it is important to control the sources of pollutants, to ventilate frequently, to change filters regularly, and to adjust humidity around 50%.

Respiratory infection such as rhinovirus or influenza infection is a major cause of asthma exacerbation and also a leading cause of the emergency room visits for asthma patients [22]. Although the prevention of respiratory infections is not always possible, washing hands is an important method of preventing the viral respiratory infection [23]. Influenza vaccination should be administered except the cases of hypersensitivity to the vaccine. Pneumococcal vaccination is also recommended [6].

7.3 Comorbid Conditions of Severe Asthma

Comorbid conditions may aggravate severe asthma by medications or by diseases themselves. Comorbid conditions may compromise treatment options as well. With the exceptions of some medications, the underlying mechanism of the relationship between comorbid conditions and severe asthma is still unclear.

Aspirin can exacerbate asthma in about 10% of asthma patients as a form of aspirin exacerbated respiratory disease (AERD) [24]. However, the prevalence of AERD increases in severe asthma up to 25% [25]. Physicians should be aware that aspirin or nonsteroidal anti-inflammatory drugs (NSAIDs) can induce very severe asthma exacerbation which could lead to intensive care unit admission or more. Aspirin or NSAIDs should be avoided in AERD. Acetaminophen can be safely used in most of the cases of AERD. Selective cyclooxygenase II inhibitors could be also considered as an alternative. But physicians should be always careful because a small portion of the patients may show hypersensitivity reactions even to acetaminophen or selective cyclooxygenase II inhibitors [26].

Beta-blocker, especially nonselective beta-blocker, should be avoided in severe asthma [27]. If necessary, selective beta1 blocker in low dose could be tried with caution. However, higher dose of selective beta1 blocker may lose the cardio-selectivity and may induce asthma exacerbation [27].

Upper airway diseases such as allergic rhinitis or sinusitis commonly coexist with asthma, which led to the concept of "one airway, one disease." Chronic rhinosinusitis is defined as an inflammatory condition in the nose and paranasal sinuses, characterized by nasal blockage or nasal discharge, in combination with facial pain/pressure or loss of smell, present for a period of at least 12 weeks [28]. Controlling rhinitis and/or sinusitis is important in the management of severe asthma [28]. Nasal saline irrigation may be helpful in addition to the use of medications such as intranasal steroid, antihistamine, and leukotriene receptor antagonist.

Gastroesophageal reflux disease may induce asthma symptoms. Avoidance of precipitating factors such as caffeine, smoking, grapefruit, and late-night eating is important as a life style modification. Medications such as proton pump inhibitors can control gastroesophageal reflux which may reduce the severity of asthma in some patients.

Weight reduction may improve asthma control as well as lung function, small airway dysfunction, and airway hyperresponsiveness [28–31]. It has been reported that severe asthma patients with obesity have more symptoms, lower lung function, and more frequent exacerbations. Obesity is also a risk factor of other comorbidities such as gastroesophageal reflux disease or obstructive sleep apnea syndrome that may aggravate asthma.

Obstructive sleep apnea syndrome is associated with poor asthma control [28, 32, 33] and is very common in severe asthma [34]. Treatment with continuous positive airway pressure may improve airway hyperresponsiveness, symptom scores, exacerbation rates, and lung function [35, 36].

Vocal cord dysfunction syndrome is caused by a paradoxical movement of the vocal cords, which induces resultant airflow limitation by the adduction of the vocal cords. The symptoms are throat tightness, stridor, hoarseness, wheezing, dyspnea, and cough, which may often lead to the misinterpretation of having severe asthma with frequent exacerbations and steroid resistance. Demonstration of paradoxical vocal cord movement is the gold standard for the diagnosis. It has been reported that the prevalence of vocal cord dysfunction syndrome is 32–50% in difficult asthma [37, 38]. Although the evidence is lacking, speech therapy that can relax vocal cords through various exercises may be helpful in the management of some severe asthma patients.

A proportion of patients with difficult asthma reports symptoms of anxiety and depression [39, 40]. It has been reported that anxiety, depression, and insomnia were associated with poor asthma control [41]. Although there is some limited evidence only, psychoeducational interventions may be helpful in the management of severe asthma with anxiety or depression.

7.4 Other Non-pharmacologic Therapies

Breathing exercise program (including physiotherapist-taught methods such as the Papworth method and the Buteyko method) could be offered to people with asthma as an adjuvant to pharmacological treatment to improve quality of life and reduce symptoms [5]. However, the evidence is limited in severe asthma.

Fish oils/lipids with n-3-polyunsaturated fatty acid, antioxidants, probiotics, acupuncture, air ionizers, and homeopathy show lack of evidence and are not recommended [5].

7.5 Future Directions

Non-pharmacological management of severe asthma consists of education, partnership, action plan, the environmental control, and the management of comorbid conditions as previously described. We are living in the era of information and communication technology such as smartphones, tablets, applications, website, social network services, computing power, and artificial intelligence. Future directions of non-pharmacological management of severe asthma are related with the advance in technology.

Smartphone and its applications could be the key components in the management of severe asthma using technology. Although severe asthma could be aggravated anytime and any-place according to the trigger factors, one cannot carry the written action plan all the time. However, smartphone is different. We bring smartphone almost everywhere and during almost all the time. Although the evidence is limited, some studies using smartphone applications on asthma management showed the possibility of increasing the adherence and improving quality of life, and of reducing systemic steroid administrations and the emergency room visits [42, 43]. Another study showed the possibility of monitoring severe asthma with geolocation and air quality [44].

There are many websites that provide useful information on asthma including the validated educational materials such as PDF files of leaflet, e-books, video clips (lecture, interview, how to use inhalers, and so on), and information on air conditions such as weather, pollen counts, and air pollution [45–47]. One problem of using websites is that patients should gain access to the website in order to acquire the materials or the information. This problem can be solved through using social network services such as Facebook, Twitter, Google+, etc. We can send these useful information via the social network services massively but specifically to the targeted users [45].

Recently studies on "Asthma Index" which predicts the possibility of asthma exacerbation have been published [48]. The Asthma Index was developed with monitoring asthma exacerbation and

possible risk factors such as temperature, common cold, air pollution, pollen counts, and so on.

Smartphone can be a platform of almost everything: education, information, partnership, and action plan. Smartphone applications that contain useful educational materials, information on the environment such as air conditions, the electronic diary on asthma that is very useful in communication and partnership with physicians, and the self-management action plans have been developed [45].

Comorbid conditions, not only disease but drug utilization, could be managed by information technology. For example, in case of aspirin or NSAIDs hypersensitivity, automatic alert can be delivered by electronic surveillance in electronic medical record system or by drug utilization review.

So far, the self-management plan on smartphone applications is based on the written action plan algorithm according to the management guidelines. Recently AlphaGo from Alphabet Inc.'s Google DeepMind became very famous after defeating the human world champions of Go [49], and IBM Watson became very famous after winning at the Jeopardy quiz show. Artificial intelligence is being studied for healthcare utilization. IBM Watson is now available for supporting the decision in the management of cancer [50]. In the near future, advance in technology may bring us in the era of managing severe asthma with artificial intelligence which may evaluate the patient's personal data including symptoms, signs, and comorbid conditions, as well as big data such as environmental risk factors simultaneously and constantly, and suggest action plans accordingly.

In conclusion, education, partnership, action plan, environmental control, management of comorbid conditions, and information technology are the essential components of non-pharmacological management in severe asthma (Fig. 7.1). Pharmacologic treatment is always important in severe asthma. However, physicians should be aware of the importance of non-pharmacological management as well. This would improve the clinical outcomes of severe asthma.

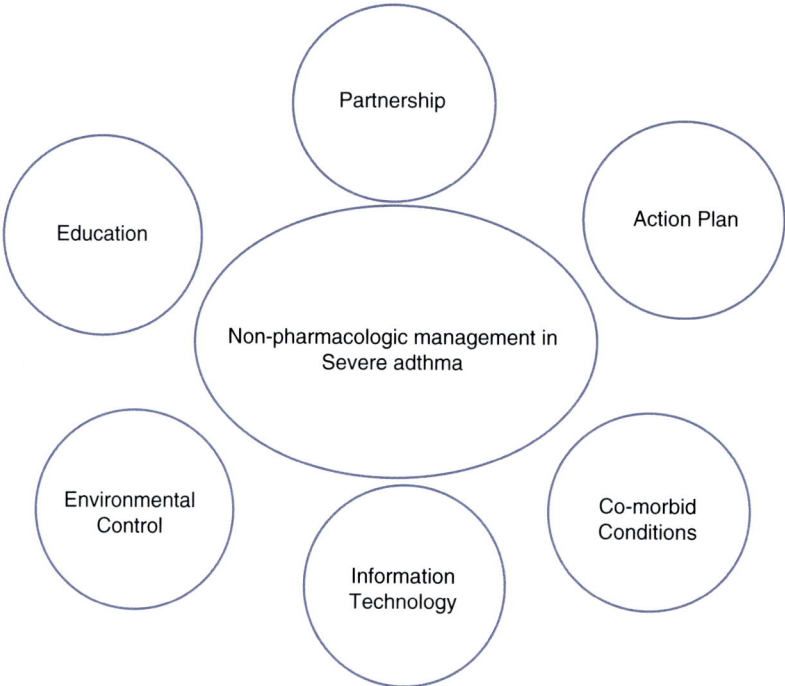

Fig. 7.1 Components of the non-pharmacological management in severe asthma

References

1. Lee SM, Chang YS, Kim CW, Kim TB, Kim SH, Kwon YE, et al. Skills in handling turbuhaler, diskus, and pressurized metered-dose inhaler in korean asthmatic patients. Allergy Asthma Immunol Res. 2011;3(1):46–52.
2. Jeong JW, Chang YS, Kim CW, Kim TB, Kim SH, Kwon YE, et al. Assessment of techniques for using inhalers in primary care physicians. Korean J Asthma Allergy Clin Immunol. 2011;31(2):116–23.
3. Kim SH, Kwak HJ, Kim TB, Chang YS, Jeong JW, Kim CW, et al. Inappropriate techniques used by internal medicine residents with three kinds of inhalers (a metered dose inhaler, Diskus, and Turbuhaler): changes after a single teaching session. J Asthma. 2009;46(9):944–50.
4. http://ginasthma.org/2017-gina-report-global-strategy-for-asthma-management-and-prevention/.
5. https://www.brit-thoracic.org.uk/document-library/clinical-information/asthma/btssign-asthma-guideline-2016/.
6. http://www.allergy.or.kr/file/150527_01.pdf.
7. Fergeson JE, Patel SS, Lockey RF. Acute asthma, prognosis, and treatment. J Allergy Clin Immunol. 2017;139(2):438–47.
8. Pawankar R, Holgate ST, Canonica GW, Lockey RF, Blaiss MS. WAO white book on allergy 2013 update. http://www.worldallergy.org/UserFiles/file/WhiteBook2-2013-v8.pdf.
9. Kim CY, Park HW, Ko SK, Chang SI, Moon HB, Kim YY, et al. The financial burden of asthma: a nationwide comprehensive survey conducted in the republic of Korea. Allergy Asthma Immunol Res. 2011;3(1):34–8.
10. Kim SH, Kim TW, Kwon JW, Kang HR, Lee YW, Kim TB, et al. Economic costs for adult asthmatics according to severity and control status in Korean tertiary hospitals. J Asthma. 2012;49(3):303–9.
11. Gotzsche PC, Johansen HK. House dust mite control measures for asthma. Cochrane Database Syst Rev. 2008;2:CD001187.
12. Fisseler-Eckhoff A, Bartsch H, Zinsky R, Schirren J. Environmental isocyanate-induced asthma: morphologic and pathogenetic aspects of an increasing occupational disease. Int J Environ Res Public Health. 2011;8(9):3672–87.
13. Park HW, Kim DI, Sohn SW, Park CH, Kim SS, Chang YS, et al. Outcomes in occupational asthma caused by reactive dye after long-term avoidance. Clin Exp Allergy. 2007;37(2):225–30.
14. Oh SS, Kim KS. Occupational asthma in Korea. J Korean Med Sci. 2010;25(Suppl):S20–5.
15. Nagasaki T, Matsumoto H. Influences of smoking and aging on allergic airway inflammation in asthma. Allergol Int. 2013;62(2):171–9.
16. Lee SY, Chang YS, Cho SH. Allergic diseases and air pollution. Asia Pac Allergy. 2013;3(3):145–54.
17. Guan WJ, Zheng XY, Chung KF, Zhong NS. Impact of air pollution on the burden of chronic respiratory

diseases in China: time for urgent action. Lancet. 2016;388(10054):1939–51.

18. Chauhan AJ, Johnston SL. Air pollution and infection in respiratory illness. Br Med Bull. 2003;68:95–112.

19. Goings SA, Kulle TJ, Bascom R, Sauder LR, Green DJ, Hebel JR, et al. Effect of nitrogen dioxide exposure on susceptibility to influenza A virus infection in healthy adults. Am Rev Respir Dis. 1989;139(5):1075–81.

20. Paulin L, Hansel N. Particulate air pollution and impaired lung function. F1000Res. 2016; 5:pii: F1000 Faculty Rev-201.

21. Watanabe M, Noma H, Kurai J, Sano H, Ueda Y, Mikami M, et al. Differences in the effects of Asian dust on pulmonary function between adult patients with asthma and those with asthma-chronic obstructive pulmonary disease overlap syndrome. Int J Chron Obstruct Pulmon Dis. 2016;11:183–90.

22. Dougherty RH, Fahy JV. Acute exacerbations of asthma: epidemiology, biology and the exacerbation-prone phenotype. Clin Exp Allergy. 2009;39(2):193–202.

23. https://www.cdc.gov/handwashing/why-handwashing.html.

24. Park SM, Park JS, Park HS, Park CS. Unraveling the genetic basis of aspirin hypersensitivity in asthma beyond arachidonate pathways. Allergy Asthma Immunol Res. 2013;5(5):258–76.

25. Ledford DK, Wenzel SE, Lockey RF. Aspirin or other nonsteroidal inflammatory agent exacerbated asthma. J Allergy Clin Immunol Pract. 2014;2(6):653–7.

26. Kim YJ, Lim KH, Kim MY, Jo EJ, Lee SY, Lee SE, et al. Cross-reactivity to acetaminophen and celecoxib according to the type of nonsteroidal anti-inflammatory drug hypersensitivity. Allergy Asthma Immunol Res. 2014;6(2):156–62.

27. Morales DR, Jackson C, Lipworth BJ, Donnan PT, Guthrie B. Adverse respiratory effect of acute β-blocker exposure in asthma: a systematic review and meta-analysis of randomized controlled trials. Chest. 2014;145(4):779–86.

28. Porsbjerg C, Menzies-Gow A. Co-morbidities in severe asthma: clinical impact and management. Respirology. 2017;22(4):651 61.

29. Dias-Junior SA, Reis M, de Carvalho-Pinto RM, Stelmach R, Halpern A, Cukier A. Effects of weight loss on asthma control in obese patients with severe asthma. Eur Respir J. 2014;43:1368–77.

30. Dixon AE, Pratley RE, Forgione PM, Kaminsky DA, Whittaker-Leclair LA, Griffes LA, et al. Effects of obesity and bariatric surgery on airway hyperresponsiveness, asthma control, and inflammation. J Allergy Clin Immunol. 2011;128:508–15.

31. Ulrik CS. Asthma and obesity. Curr Opin Pulm Med. 2016;22:69–73.

32. Tay TR, Radhakrishna N, Hore-Lacy F, Smith C, Hoy R, Dabscheck E, et al. Comorbidities in difficult asthma are independent risk factors for frequent exacerbations, poor control and diminished quality of life. Respirology. 2016;21:1384–90.

33. Teodorescu M, Broytman O, Curran-Everett D, Sorkness RL, Crisafi G, Bleecker ER, et al. Obstructive sleep apnea risk, asthma burden, and lower airway inflammation in adults in the Severe Asthma Research Program (SARP) II. J Allergy Clin Immunol Pract. 2015;3:566–75.

34. Julien JY, Martin JG, Ernst P, Olivenstein R, Hamid Q, Lemière C, et al. Prevalence of obstructive sleep apnea–hypopnea in severe versus moderate asthma. J Allergy Clin Immunol. 2009;124:371–6.

35. Serrano-Pariente J, Plaza V, Soriano JB, Mayos M, López-Viña A, Picado C, Vigil L, CPASMA Trial Group. Asthma outcomes improve with continuous positive airway pressure for obstructive sleep apnea. Allergy. 2017;72:802–12. doi:10.1111/all.13070.

36. Busk M, Busk N, Puntenney P, Hutchins J, Yu Z, Gunst SJ, et al. Use of continuous positive airway pressure reduces airway reactivity in adults with asthma. Eur Respir J. 2013;41:317–22.

37. Tay TR, Radhakrishna N, Hore-Lacy F, Smith C, Hoy R, Dabscheck E, et al. Comorbidities in difficult asthma are independent risk factors for frequent exacerbations, poor control and diminished quality of life. Respirology. 2016;21:1384–90.

38. Low K, Lau KK, Holmes P, Crossett M, Vallance N, Phyland D, et al. Abnormal vocal cord function in difficult-to-treat asthma. Am J Respir Crit Care Med. 2011;184:50–6.

39. von Bülow A, Kriegbaum M, Backer V, Porsbjerg C. The prevalence of severe asthma and low asthma control among Danish adults. J Allergy Clin Immunol Pract. 2014;2:759–67.

40. Haldar P, Pavord ID, Shaw DE, Berry MA, Thomas M, Brightling CE, et al. Cluster analysis and clinical asthma phenotypes. Am J Respir Crit Care Med. 2008;178:218–24.

41. Luyster FS, Strollo PJ Jr, Holguin F, Castro M, Dunican EM, Fahy J, et al. Association between insomnia and asthma burden in the Severe Asthma Research Program (SARP) III. Chest. 2016;15:1242–50.

42. Kim MY, Lee SY, Jo EJ, Lee SE, Kang MG, Song WJ, et al. Feasibility of a smartphone application based action plan and monitoring in asthma. Asia Pac Allergy. 2016;6(3):174–80.

43. Kim BY, Lee J. Smart devices for older adults managing chronic disease: a scoping review. JMIR Mhealth Uhealth. 2017;5(5):e69.

44. Chan YY, Wang P, Rogers L, Tignor N, Zweig M, Hershman SG, et al. The Asthma Mobile Health Study, a large-scale clinical observational study using ResearchKit. Nat Biotechnol. 2017;35(4):354–62.

45. http://e-allergy.org.

46. https://www.nationalasthma.org.au.

47. http://allergypot.net.

48. Yun HS, Rah WJ, Choi YJ, Kim JH, Oh JW, Kim HH, et al. The development of patient-tailored asthma prediction model for the alarm system. Allergy Asthma Respir Dis. 2016;4(5):328–39.

49. https://en.wikipedia.org/wiki/AlphaGo.

50. https://en.wikipedia.org/wiki/Watson_(computer).

Index

A

Air pollution, 125
Air trapping in asthma, 91
Airway remodeling, 37–40
    activated fibroblasts/myofibroblasts, 37
    ASM, 39
    asthmatic severity, 37
    bronchial epithelium, 37, 38
    ECM alterations, 40
    epithelial changes, 37
    smooth muscle mass, 37
    subepithelial fibrosis, 37, 40
    subepithelial thickening, 40
    vascular changes, 37
    vascular remodeling, 40
Airway smooth muscle (ASM), 39
Airway wall thickening, 92
Allergic bronchopulmonary aspergillosis
    (ABPA), 8, 9, 23, 110
    airway hypersensitivity, fungi, 19
    Aspergillus sensitization, 22
    Aspergillus spore, 20
    classification, 21
    clinical features, 21
    complications, 20
    diagnostic criteria, 21, 22
    differential diagnosis, 19, 21
    histologic features, 21, 23
    histological methods, 20
    immediate skin reactivity, 22
    management, 23
    pathogenesis, 20, 21
    prevalence, 20
    pulmonary opacities, 22
    serum eosinophilia, 22
    spirometry, 22
    stages, 21
    treatment, 20
        acute exacerbations, 23
        antifungal therapy, 23
        glucocorticosteroids, 23
        omalizumab, 23
        voriconazole, 23
Allergic bronchopulmonary mycosis (ABPM), 8
Allergic rhinitis, 18
Antifungal agents, 10
Anti-IgE monoclonal antibody (mAb), 104, 105
Anti-interleukin (IL)-5 monoclonal antibody, 5
Anti-interleukins, 109
Antioxidants, 47, 103
Anti-tumor necrosis factor α (TNF-α), 109
Arachidonic acid metabolites, 67
Aspirin-exacerbated respiratory disease (AERD), 18, 125
    aspirin desensitization, 26, 27
    diagnosis, 24, 25
    management, 26
    mechanism of, 25
    medications, 26
    nonallergic induced asthma, 24
    pathogenesis, 25, 27
    prevalence, 24
    surgical approach, 27
    symptoms, 24
Asthma Index, 127
Asthma Predictive Index (API), 73
Asthma-COPD overlap syndrome (ACOS)
    definition, 13
    diagnosis and treatment, 14, 15
    epidemiology, 14
    management, 15
    prevalence, 14
    treatment approaches, 15
Asthmatic airway epithelium, 38
Atelectasis, 90

B

Blood
    adhesion molecules, 70
    cytokines and growth factors, 70

Printed in the United States
By Bookmasters